1.69

WHY

- does an apple a day *really* help keep the doctor away?
- are citrus fruits—"golden sunshine"—best eaten with caution—if at all?
- do you keep getting colds, feeling tired or depressed?
- is a natural supplement preferable to a synthetic?
- is sugar a prime danger to your body and mind?
- is fiber one of the most vital of the body's needs— yet steadily disappearing from your diet?
- should you have at least one fermented food a day?

These are questions you may never have thought of asking—yet the answers can affect your health for the rest of your life.

Calling for the achievement and maintenance of bodily health by natural means rather than the standard treatment of individual symptoms as they arise, PREVENTIVE ORGANIC MEDICINE instructs the reader in how the body and its systems operate and shows how natural nutrition functions in assuring its best possible condition—the radiant good health we all want and are entitled to.

PREVENTIVE ORGANIC MEDICINE

Your Passport to Good Health

by KURT W. DONSBACH, D.C., N.D.

Keats Publishing, Inc.
New Canaan, Connecticut

Compiled by JOHN LOUIS FRIES
Illustrations by Jim Lentine

Preventive Organic Medicine,
Your Passport to Good Health

Pivot edition published 1976 by Keats Publishing, Inc.

Copyright © 1972, 1976 by Kurt W. Donsbach, D.C., N.D.

Library of Congress Catalog Number: 76-2979

Printed in the United States of America

Keats Publishing, Inc.
36 Grove Street (Box 876)
New Canaan, Connecticut 06840

CONTENTS

FOREWORD

The book you are about to read will speak for itself; I am indeed grateful for the opportunity of adding a few brief paragraphs about the author, a devoted humanitarian steadfast in his dedication to helping people obtain good health through proper nutrition.

The Doctor and I met in 1962. At the time, I was extremely ill and fatigued, existing almost solely on tranquilizers and in a deep state of depression. I was well acquainted with the medical profession at the time, as an owner of rest homes and sanitariums; still, I was unable to find the answer to my continuing and declining health problems. Then, Kurt took me under his wing! His advice and nutritional expertise soon combined to make me well and whole again. Careful selection of the right foods and menus, exercise and an adequate supplementation program reversed my downsliding health pattern and I suddenly discovered what "feeling good" was like once again.

A word of caution! After reading this book, do not expect instantaneous results. Anything worth doing is worth doing well and that includes a Preventive Organic Medicine Program. I vividly recall the passage of at least two weeks time before I experienced any feeling of improvement at all. In fact, by the end of the first week I remember actually feeling worse rather than better as the toxins began departing my system.

Does Preventive Organic Medicine really work? I recently saw friends I had not seen for years; they were literally amazed at my appearance, remarking I looked ten years younger than I did at our last meeting ten years earlier. That has to be proof positive when you are speaking of a lady almost—but not quite—at the half century mark!

It has been a delightful almost-half century— and a healthy one these past years. It is my hope and prayer that my husband, through these pages, will be able to help you live longer naturally and in better health through Preventive Organic Medicine.

Elyse Donsbach

ACKNOWLEDGMENTS

In writing this book I do not intend to take original credit for its contents. I have borrowed liberally from many great men who have preceded me in this fascinating study of the human body and its inherent ability to heal itself if we but try to understand and assist biochemical changes.

Special credit belongs to my wife Elyse for her constant insistence that this work should be completed; to Dr. Marion Loftin, Salt Lake City, for his wise counsel in my beginning efforts as a writer; to Dr. Royal Lee, Milwaukee, for his inspiration and constant example in the years I knew and worked with him; to John Louis Fries, Garden Grove, California for his able assistance in compiling and editing this work; and to the many, many friends who have made known their desire for a book of this nature.

INTRODUCTION

About a million years ago, modern man sprang from the roots of simple origins with primitive habits and facilities. Today we walk on the moon and man-made vehicles journey in the shadows of Venus and Mars.

Primitive man could probably not have eaten unwisely if he tried. His problem then was getting enough food to stave off hunger. Modern man, however, has great difficulty selecting foods for a proper and balanced diet. Our problem is the overabundance of food upon which we tend to stuff.

Modern man has even set up a timetable schedule of eating and given it a label—"three square meals a day." Eating habits should be regulated by hunger, not custom, to generate good health and well-being. Brillat Savarin, the famous French gourmet and politician put it succinctly: "An animal swallows its food, a man eats it, but only a man of intellect knows how to dine."

We can not imagine any knowledgeable person sitting down to a table cluttered with garbage and dirt and infested with flies and insects. Yet many supposedly intelligent and charming people think nothing of eating all sorts of pasty, gooey, dampening, souring kinds of foods which interfere with intestinal hygiene. This is shameful! A really healthful, sweet and wholesome intestinal environment is literally impossible under such circumstances. And, to make matters worse, a majority of our citizens have not the slightest knowledge of what this kind of abuse does to them, or what they can do about it.

The field of assisting the ailments of the human body is one of the most intriguing and engrossing studies possible. The history of the various approaches to healing is a turmoil of correct and incorrect theories, liberally laced with politics, social status and, at times, out-and-out profiteering. This book is not intended to credit or discredit any approach to healing; it is designed to set forth a theory that the human body with its innate intelligence can, with the help of a rational, common sense, conscious intelligence, be free from disease as we now know it.

A "Passport to Good Health" is readily yours, but your journey will not necessarily be easy. You will undoubtedly come to the conclusion after reviewing this work, that your common sense could have told you most of what it contains. To "validate" your passport, of course, will require conscious, daily adherence to the basic laws of nature, in your nutritional intake and proper exercise and your own personal instinct of survival. With all the social, political and ecological problems of a changing and complex world, stormy waters are certain to engulf you as you sail upon the turbulent sea of a healthy productive life.

In this regard, it is my studied conviction that the entire practice of medicine (including all the various approaches used to assist the body toward a more healthful existence) is just that—a practice—a theory—definitely not a science in the accepted form of the word.

One of the major criteria for a science involves irrefutable rules—rules which say that one plus one will always equal two. In working with the human body there are too many variables for such rigid rules; all the variables must be taken into consideration before any answers are realized. One plus one may equal zero or five, depending on various factors, when the extremely complex body chemical mechanism is involved.

Because of these variables (which many times become imponderables), I have attempted to set forth a concept free from prejudice which in practical application could be a system of caring for the human body without the use of harsh drugs. It must be strictly understood that I have every respect for the surgeon who adds precious years with open heart surgery or who repairs a mangled limb into a useful part of the body. His consummate skill has benefited countless recipients and is much to be admired.

We hope that our theory—Preventive Organic Medicine through the proper use of nature's own elements, nutritional guidelines, physical activity and a positive, moral state of mind—will gain increased momentum in the coming years. As in so many endeavors, we have but to journey back in time to realize the wisdom of the ages. Good health, today as in biblical times, is a state of mind and with ample adherence to the rules of good nutrition, hygiene and exercise, can rapidly become the norm for us all. Remember, paying attention to preventive medicine is the surest way to "cure what *does not* ail you."

Now, read on, dear reader—

your "Passport to Good Health" awaits you!

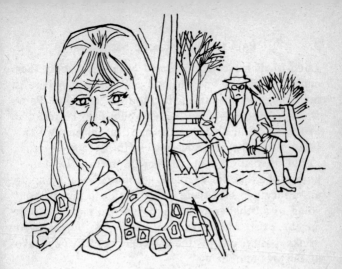

Chapter 1

"I WISH I WERE DEAD"

HOW OFTEN I have heard the words "I wish I were dead," uttered dejectedly by a person seriously ill and in the depths of despair. Usually, all modes of treatment have long been exhausted with apparently little or no hope left.

It is incongruous to me that in this day of advanced scientific endeavor, financed by billions upon billions of research dollars every year, the physical and mental health of the human species continues to slide and decline let alone show any signs of relief. It would give me great pleasure to be able to say to these inflicted and suffering masses: "Have hope, I have a panacea for you which will take care of all your problems."

Unfortunately, this is not possible, as the burden of improvement always rests on the shoulders of the individuals themselves. If the philosophy of Preventive Or-

1

ganic Medicine could suddenly be grasped, only then could I truthfully and in good conscience say there is hope and good health in the future of mankind. Pain-wracked, disease-ridden bodies would then be restored to their rightful places as the most magnificently functioning organisms ever designed by the Creator.

But that poses yet another problem. "Doctor, I haven't the time for exercise, nutritional meal planning and education. Isn't there something I can take without going to all that trouble? And you really can't expect me to exist without coffee, cigarettes, liquor, soft drinks, pastry, etc. [as the case may be]; it would take all the joy out of living."

I tactfully remind these people that if they really enjoyed the fruits of such a life they would not be in my office seeking help. Then an air of injured martyrdom becomes apparent: "Doctor, if you can promise to make me well, I will do and try anything!" Of course, what is really meant is that if the patient is feeling better after the first day or two of treatment, the doctor is regarded as a modern day miracle worker. But if the problem persists for a few days without noticeable results, the patient quickly reverts back to his same old, self-defeating habits of the past. This basic nature of man, whether it be shown in his quest for fortune or for good health, is responsible for that feeling of quiet frustration that often manifests itself in otherwise competent, capable doctors. I can not help but marvel at the wonderful patience and indulgence demonstrated by these men; I often wonder if perhaps certain facets and traits of ministerial training should not be part of the educational process, in particular for the professions.

The basic instinct of every dedicated doctor is to relieve suffering wherever it may be. In order to accomplish this without producing or inflicting other pains or side effects, nature must be considered and measures taken to maintain that balance so necessary to good health and long life. It has always been the philosophy of practitioners of Preventive Organic Medicine that only under the most severe circumstances should drugs or drastic surgery be resorted to. Drugs are inert substances which can produce a violent reaction in the body because of toxicity and are entirely against the plan of nature, being neither intrinsically healing nor beneficial. On the other hand, natural elements are living substances that exert a structural, building effect on the body and are the basis of good, sound Preventive Organic Medicine.

THE BASIS OF DISEASE

As a general practitioner of naturopathic and chiropractic methods of healing since 1957, I have successfully treated all manner of diseases, acute and chronic. To be a real physician in every sense of the word, I have found it imperative to utilize every method of healing available including the inspired healing powers of divine faith and an uncompromising belief in a Supreme Being. We may all be brothers under the sun, but as individuals, we all differ from one another physically, mentally and in dietary needs. We must even utilize different suggestive techniques. Some patients will respond to one approach, while others can only be reached by way of a completely different avenue. For that reason, new methods and solutions must constantly be sought, with the results and experience thus gained made available to others for the maximum benefit of all mankind.

THE ONE BASIC DISEASE

It is my opinion, based on many years of research and practical experience, that there is but one basic disease—*toxemia*. Consider a healthy individual to whom a thousand and one things can happen to bring his physical and mental condition below normal. He may receive physical or mental shock which interferes with his metabolism. He may overeat, worry or do any of the innumerable things which will lower his stamina and energy level. Soon, tension develops that interferes with digestion and elimination and a gradual accumulation of toxins in the body takes place. These poisons are composed of retained normal waste products, toxic substances which have failed to be detoxified by the body, absorbed toxic products of abnormal digestion and toxins constantly in the environment which we daily battle to eliminate or isolate from our vital organs.

It seems to be modern man's basic inclination to actually resist, either actively or passively, nature's attempts to maintain good health. If Madison Avenue cries: "Try it—you'll like it," we become convinced it is perfectly proper to overeat to the point of discomfort because a quick, painless remedy is at hand to alleviate the problem with the trickle of a fizzle. How much better to treat the cause—overindulgence—rather than the symptom—upset stomach or indigestion—by practicing Preventive Organic Medicine. There can be little doubt such a departure from current custom would severely curtail the American economy, if we paid more attention to the cause and stopped pampering the symptoms of so-called disease. Think of the thousands and thousands of patent remedies that would simply go begging if only nature was allowed to do the job without interference, and without undue influence from advertising copywriters. Instead of resorting to pain killers and tranquilizers, let us try to find the cause of our discomfort and remove it. Mother Nature will do the rest!

TREAT THE CAUSE—NOT THE SYMPTOM

Television, radio, magazines, newspapers, et al, have taught and encouraged people by clever ads and easy slogans to depend upon relief instead of removing the cause. As a result, our hospitals are full and runneth over. In an article in *Pageant* magazine, the statement was made: "We do live longer—but we disintegrate faster. In this country there are hundreds of thousands of people in State Hospitals for the insane with many thousands more being admitted every year." Why? The answer is obvious.

The majority of us eat at least three times as much food daily as the body requires to maintain health. All food eaten in excess of body requirements increases the chances of arthritis, indigestion and other disease symptoms. In my office one day, I overheard one patient tell another, "It's funny, the less I eat the better I feel and I just can't understand it."

People have been taught to eat to keep up their strength for so many years that it comes as a shock to learn they have been misinformed. Eating to maintain strength during illness has eliminated more human life than any other one thing. A man trying to get over a spell of the flu told a friend if he could just eat he knew he would be all right. He associated a good appetite with a good feeling. Had he used his good old-fashioned horse sense, he would have realized that a horse, even a slow one, will not eat when sick. Nor will any other animal; the human animal is the only one who insists on eating when not well.

People have been taught from birth to eat and eat and eat. When an infant has fever and you offer it milk, the baby invariably will accept it. What parents or nurses do not seem to understand is the baby will take water just as readily because, in reality, it is thirsty, not hungry. When a person is running a fever, it is a sure sign the body is trying to burn up toxins in the blood. Food of any kind should be withheld; it matters not what you think caused the fever.

An old Chinese proverb states: "If you stuff a cold, you will have to starve a fever later." But people do not like the idea of going without food for a few meals so they reverse the saying to: "Stuff a cold; starve a fever." For instance, parents consistently insist on stuffing childhood colds with all kinds of patent remedies and solutions, but completely ignore the necessity of starving the fever to eliminate the cause. As a result, the fever is suppressed and temporary relief sometimes received, but the child is sentenced to carry certain toxins in his body to adulthood. Invariably, in time such toxins will manifest themselves as symptoms of some chronic disease and we curse the cruel fates that brought a loved one to such an untimely and tragic end.

When a person complains he has not felt well since he suffered a bad case of the flu some time back, he is really telling you he was never cured of the cause; his symptoms were merely suppressed and cloaked under a blanket of unnatural remedies. Few if any patients of allopathic medicine are allowed to recover *naturally*. Quick pain killers to suppress symptoms are insisted upon; then, if we feel even slightly improved, we just let it go at that.

The efforts of nature are always directed toward keeping life in the body as long as possible, even if in modified or reduced form. If the body becomes diseased, it must be cleansed of debris, not burdened with extraneous and nonproductive food to be digested and processed by the same ailing system. If this simple but vital lesson would be heeded, the medical and hospital bills of most American families would be slashed tremendously. Even more important, it would alleviate untold misery and needless suffering on this earth.

DIAGNOSIS AND THERAPY

The body is composed of untold millions of minute organized cells which are grouped together into functional entities known as organs. Studies of disease in the human organism have been made primarily by means of tests of blood, urine, feces, and saliva, tests which are not studies of the cells themselves. The action and growth, i.e., the physiology, of cells themselves has barely been explored. Yet we diagnose disease from a level far removed from the basic structure of life in the human form (the cell), and then attempt to treat and improve life-giving functions from such meager and possibly misleading secretions.

An organ of the body consists of any part of the body having a specialized function. Each organ consists of innumerable, complex cells. Microscopic examination of an organ tissue can readily reveal tissue damage but does not reveal what the functional disturbance actually is.

Therefore, when any therapeutic or diagnostic method is employed, it is at the organ level, not the cellular level. When we speak of the heart, for example, we refer to it as an organ. Our evaluation of its reaction to any therapeutic agent is based upon the total cooperative effect of numberless heart tissue cells.

Diagnostically, there is no known method of determining the status of the cells as individuals or as separate entities. And, of course, it is upon these cells that the total activity of the organ depends.

This observation of function in the subject is referred to as empirical medicine—based upon the skill and observation of the physician. When considered from this viewpoint, practically all therapeutic and diagnostic methods used today depend upon empirical medicine; that is to say, the acid test still remains in the "crucible of the clinic."

As a clinician, the physician has two primary therapeutic possibilities to consider. First, those therapeutic means which are normally present in the body, namely, those provided by the food, air and water intake and commonly referred to as nutrition; secondly, those things not normally found in the body and foreign to its economy, which we call drugs.

In observing the action of these drugs as they affect the organs of the body, we have a comparatively simple task. For example, the action of digitalis (or almost any other drug) is quite obvious and conspicuous. The reaction by organs is quite easily observed.

However, in studying the action of nutritional entities, we find just the opposite situation. A clear picture of their effects is very difficult to bring into focus because nutrients act at the cellular level and do not always reflect an immediate change at the organ level.

Under certain conditions the nutritional approach to therapy may have just as dramatic a response as the drug approach, but more often than not, the total effect is much slower. Nutritional help, nevertheless, is an active and corrective additive from the moment it is introduced into the body to offset any deficiency present. Its effects are immediate; there is nothing to impair the reactivity of the organ concerned. This type of action is completely opposite to a drug reaction which has no immediate dynamic or positive effect on the cell, but must wait for the reaction of the cells to a foreign substance. This reaction may be either inhibitory or stimulative in its effect.

The medical arts employ drugs to a great degree and as a basic facet of the profession. As students and observers of drug effects, physicians, nurses and technicians have become proficient and knowledgeable. One should realize that the tremendous respect and awe tendered the medical profession by the public is to no small degree based upon this proficiency. On the other hand, these same medical practitioners are severely limited in extending their astute observatory powers to the nutritional field—which requires a much more subtle insight into effects—by the requirements of so-called orthodoxy, which decrees that a specific drug must be used in a certain circumstance to achieve a particular reaction or result.

One thing is rather obvious—the physician who limits himself to drug therapy is playing it safe. Present-day laws and practice protect the orthodox physician regardless of the consequences to the patient. On the other hand, the dedicated and inquisitive physician who delves into the unknown (even though his methods be thoroughly qualified as to their safety, by reason of being normal and natural to the human organisms) is considered unorthodox and is liable to persecution—legal persecution. Certainly, the situation does not revolve around which is right and which is wrong. In one case, drug therapy may be necessary to save a life, whereas in another case, drug therapy may not be indicated and nutritional support would be best for the welfare of the patient.

The real issue is the right of the physician to act in the interest of the patient as he is qualified by education, as against the right of the individual to choose whatever means he wishes to regain, protect or maintain his health. No person should be allowed to interfere with this personal and God-given right nor should any law or ordinance be enacted which shall abrogate or deny such a right. It is not a matter of "the consensus of medical opinion," but rather of the individual's right to act as his "own man" instead of having someone else do his thinking for him under the guise of "big brother" or "father knows best."

A good example of this situation is a patient with a heart condition for which the standard orthodox medical treatment is the administration of digitalis. The patient, not benefited by this approach, seeks another medical doctor. Diagnosis and prescription are the same. The patient is bewildered! He has had two competent medical opinions, both concurring, but his basic problem remains the same. Does he not have the right, both legally and morally, to seek an unorthodox approach to his problem in order to secure relief and regain his failing health?

This is by no means an indictment of the practice of allopathic medicine. People are satisfactorily relieved of acute symptoms every day by this approach to the disease problem. What we would like to point out at this particular time is the divergence of approach available to the healing profession, and the uncontested fact that no one philosophy has a monopoly on knowledge.

TO HEAL IS NATURAL—TO CURE DIVINE

Preventive Organic Medicine is a complete system of healing based on the study of health and how to promote it. This system embraces the use of nature's agen-

cies, forces, processes and products according to the indications of the individual.

BASIC PREMISE

The basic premise of Preventive Organic Medicine is
that the human body is self-curing when it functions
properly; therefore, the duty of the physician is to promote normal function. The procedure is to determine
first how, why and to what extent a given body has
deviated from normal function. This is accomplished
by evaluating the objective and subjective symptoms.
Objective symptoms, of course, are the outward signs
which can be observed, such as appearance, behavior,
structural distortions and results of laboratory tests.
Subjective symptoms are the abnormal sensations of
which the individual is aware.

Corrective procedures are, in my opinion, two-fold
in nature: (1) Restoration to normalcy of the biochemistry in general, and (2) Care of the localized
symptoms.

As noted, the primary consideration is to normalize
the biochemistry of the body and not to treat the symptomatic picture as does the doctor of allopathic medicine.

The corrective procedures in this regard can be categorized as follows: (1) Eliminate excess waste products from the blood and lymphatic circulation; (2)
Supply the elements to nourish tissues; (3) Restore
physiological harmony between interrelated systems
such as glandular and nerve functions, structural and
muscular coordination and the function of digestion
and elimination; (4) Promote mental and emotional
tranquility.

In all fairness, it should be noted that some of the
procedures used in accomplishing the first objective

also accomplish the second objective, namely relieving symptoms. Some of the methods used in this manner are massage, manipulation, fasting, controlled diet, concentrated supplementation of nutritional factors, hydrotherapy, electrotherapy and other physical and physiotherapy adjuncts.

The foregoing is the basic premise of Preventive Organic Medicine. This, however, is overshadowed by the far more important factors of philosophy and principles, for it is only from these two factors that understanding and acceptance can come about.

Organic medicine is preventive as well as curative. Health and disease are opposites, much as light and darkness; in order to dissipate darkness, it is but necessary to increase light. In a similar manner we need but to institute measures that tend to improve general body activity in order to modify any diseased condition. After it has been determined why the body has ceased to function properly, the correct methods can be applied to restore normal activity and the body then becomes self-curing.

FACTORS TO CONSIDER

Since the body constantly renews itself, it will deviate from normal only when it is chemically out of balance or when it is in an unsuitable environment. Both of these factors, then, must be considered. Chemically out of balance means that we have too much of some elements and not enough of others; an unsuitable environment may mean too hot, too cold, too wet, too dry, etc.

Disease is the result of impaired function. Symptoms are due to the body's efforts to adjust itself to a change in environment. A diagnosed disease process is the final manifestation of the body's functional deviation from normal. The subject is aware of effects only and not of causes.

The mental and emotional aspects must also be considered. That is, we must ascertain what effects anxieties may have on a given problem or in what way indifference may interfere with normalizing procedures under certain circumstances. This is why the competent doctor must be capable in the field of applied psychology as well as medicine.

Life has been defined as a continuous adjustment to a constantly changing environment. This applies to every individual cell in the body as well as to the body as a whole. So, we must begin with the single cell and then proceed to the various organs and parts of the body. Eventually, we reach the several interrelated systems such as the circulatory, digestive, eliminative and lymphatic systems. Finally, we study the body as a whole including mental and emotional activity. Removing waste products from the tissues is tantamount to changing the environment of the individual cell to which it must adjust itself. A change in diet or the addition of nutritional supplements also will alter cell environment to which the cell must adjust.

INITIAL STEPS

The process of normalizing function is begun by eliminating waste products from the tissues which change the environment of every cell in the body. This is followed by making any needed change in the diet and, in most instances, adding in supplemental form those elements of nutrition found to be deficient. This creates yet a further change in cellular environment. By this process, it is found that cell adjustment is toward normal, whereas, when certain toxic drugs are used to change cell environment, the adjustment is away from the normal.

The foregoing procedures are followed in all cases except those of injuries or other emergencies. Now that you are familiar with Preventive Organic Medicine, let us compare our philosophy with that of allopathic medicine. (You will note that the word "medicine" is used in the connotation of the healing art and not to mean allopathic philosophy as commonly accepted.) For example, let us examine the procedures in treating a patient whose stomach is ulcerated. In ulceration, tissue cells are breaking down faster than they are replaced. Organic medicine directs its efforts to establishing chemical balance by assisting the body in the elimination of metabolic residue or waste products from the tissues and by supplying the materials necessary to rebuild deteriorated linings. Palliative measures may be used for a short time to give relief from severe, acute symptoms until the restorative procedure becomes effective. The patient is instructed to proceed with a normal balanced diet quite early in the treating process. Prognosis for recovery is most favorable.

ORTHODOX METHOD

Orthodox allopathic medicine in a similar case usually directs its efforts toward obliterating the patient's symptoms by prescribing a bland diet and perhaps antacids. The *Merck Manual* (the allopathic guide book) states that other types of medications are administered to coat the gastric and intestinal linings to protect from irritation by normal acids. In many cases, however, the ulcerating tissue cells continue to degenerate until surgery becomes necessary or the patient develops even more serious problems. Prognosis is poor; recovery is usually slow and uncertain.

Another patient may complain of feeling weak and nervous. In all probability this individual has been examined by several physicians and told, "There's nothing wrong with you, you're just nervous." The doctor of organic medicine finds that these cases usually improve under simple procedures of cleansing the lymphatic and blood systems and improving nutrition. It has been amply demonstrated over the years that deficiencies of certain mineral elements can contribute much toward a nervous attitude. Prognosis is usually very good when nature is employed as the healing element.

The allopath often prescribes for prolonged, indefinite periods a glandular hormone or its derivative. Sometimes caffeine (or a similar medication) to relieve the feeling of weakness, and a barbiturate to subdue the nervous symptoms are utilized. This is orthodox procedure according to the much used and heralded *Merck Manual.* New and at times controversial tranquilizers are also being used in great quantity by "progressive" allopaths to control nervous symptoms. With this approach, the possibility of addiction should not be overlooked. The prognosis in such cases is more times than not unfavorable with little hope for improvement awaiting the unfortunate and misguided recipient.

"DOCTOR, HOW LONG WILL IT TAKE?"

The question most doctors like to avoid is: "How long will it be until I am well again?" It is a question so loaded with variables that no human could possibly predict the answer with any degree of certainty. The most critical part of the problem lies in the individual himself. Some patients follow instructions with precision and with the proper mental attitude. Others are slipshod and rebellious, quickly adopting the attitude the doctor is unjustifiably taking precious little "vices" away by recommending a cleansing diet or abstinence from cigarettes, coffee or alcohol.

TWO WEEKS, IF ...

I have, over a period of years, come to the conclusion that most conditions can be symptomatically relieved to such an extent that the patient is aware of the changes within two weeks if certain rules of conduct are obediently followed. There are physicians who will throw up their hands upon reading this and say, "Impossible!" That, of course, is their prerogative; I am confident that upon analyzing my methods and the reasons for them, you will see the logic and feasibility of such a contention.

My premise is based on the indisputable fact that all people ill with physical and/or mental problems are congested with toxins in their system, either in the blood stream, the liver or the digestive tract. This congestion may be relieved by rather simple measures if we possess information as to which means should be used to release the toxins from the particular area involved.

Unfortunately, the simple remedies are often the most difficult to master because of their very simplicity. If a patient receives a horrendous-sounding diagnosis and is also given dangerous medication to "try" to overcome his condition, he usually is satisfied that his money has been well-spent whether he recovers good health or not. On the other hand, if a patient uses a herb solution such as yerba santa to overcome a lung congestion of several months' standing and is not well overnight, he often complains that the herbal did not work and discontinues its use. Because yerba santa does not have the approval of orthodox medicine, it is not always used with the wholehearted enthusiasm necessary to give any remedy a proper chance. A point to remember, then, is that the remedy, once decided upon, should be used with confidence and enthusiasm.

BASIC DIFFERENCE

To sum up the basic difference between allopathic and organic medicine, let me make a comparison. On one side of the fence, we have a philosophy which tries to destroy or stifle the intruder supposedly responsible for the condition of the body (disease); on the other side, we have that philosophy dedicated to cleansing and restoring to normal the inner environment of the patient on the premise that a normal, healthy body cannot countenance disease.

There is yet another issue to be considered in this discussion, and that issue is a moral one. It is undesirable, unreasonable, inhuman and intolerable to think of permitting one school of thought to dominate all others in the field of medicine (again, "medicine" refers to all the healing arts) and to be given final authority in all matters pertaining to health. Health is an individual's most priceless possession. A violation of individual conscience on the subject of health can have the most far-reaching and devastating effect.

It is declared a noble and time-honored condition in this country that no one has the right to deny another the right to life, liberty and the pursuit of happiness. Logically, then, it must follow that it is immoral and imprudent to deny anyone the right and freedom to choose whatever he may feel to be adequate and desirable in solving his own health problems. To be or not to be healthy is a question that should be answered only by the individual involved, according to the dictates of personal conscience and subject only to the higher realm of the Almighty.

For almost 2,000 years, allopathic medicine has controlled the healing arts almost the world over. In certain areas in our own United States, there are laws which make the practice of any form of healing except that of allopathic medicine a felony. Such a situation is loathsome and decadent and certainly not in keeping with progressive and open-minded thinking. Thomas Jefferson once said, "I know of no safe depository of the ultimate powers of society but the people themselves; and if we think them not enlightened enough to exercise their control with a wholesome discretion, the remedy is not to take it from them, but to inform their discretion by education." It is unfortunate that the great majority of educational programs made available for public consumption regarding the healing arts are almost entirely prepared and released by the self-serving, public relations arm of the allopath—the American Medical Association. Public officials and legislators alike are bombarded continuously and unrelentingly by the AMA with copious, self-oriented, one-sided arguments supporting and actively promoting the allopathic approach to medicine as the only true and feasible solution to the age-old problem of disease and relief from pain.

It is an understatement of fact to state that allopathic medicine is extremely vulnerable to the charge of insensitivity to other methods of healing. Sir William Osler, M.D. (1849-1919), conceded to be the foremost authority on drugs in his day and whose teaching and personality have strongly influenced medical progress (physician-in-chief, Johns Hopkins Hospital, Baltimore [1889-1905] and professor of medicine, Johns Hopkins University; regius professor of medicine [1905-1919], Oxford University, England), expressed my sentiments exactly when he said: "We use drugs about which we know little in a body about which we know less to cure disease about which we know nothing at all."

Many times the piously offered allopathic cure has turned out to be much worse for the patient than the so-called disease. Thank God for Nature—and her "Passport to Good Health" which can be validated anywhere on this good earth if only we take the time and trouble to play our part.

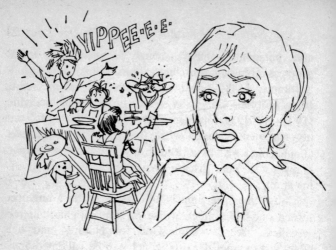

Chapter II

CAN NUTRITION AFFECT STRESS OF MODERN-DAY LIFE?

ALAS, WE hear it every day! Patients say, "I'm a bundle of nerves! Little things tire me; children bother me; noise upsets me. I wish I could relax! Why can't I sleep any more?"

The number of ways the patient can find to express extra-excitability—commonly called jittery nerves or heebie-jeebies—is almost endless. In this day and age it is a common complaint and can be difficult to treat if the patient is not aware of some of the contributing factors.

Let's take a simile to illustrate the situation. If "regular" gas is used in a high compression engine, when

20

the ignition switch is turned off the motor may fail to stop immediately and continue to idle. Changing to high-test fuel corrects the difficulty. The same is true of people complaining of nervousness. When the time comes for them to relax they can not "turn off" and the effects of stimulation which should abate, continue. Environmental stimuli take on exaggerated proportions.

This particular condition is not in itself a disease. It may only mean that the "fuel" necessary to a balanced nervous system is of the wrong grade. This also explains why on certain days the excitability pattern is more exaggerated than on other days. The "fuel" which we refer to is, of course, furnished by the food we eat. It has been well established that certain nutrients have the ability to desensitize the person who has been deficient in them.

Our everyday living habits are sometimes so rushed that we rarely bother to consider the fact that our body is the finest and most precise piece of machinery known to man. Certainly it deserves a bit of attention as to the "fuel" which keeps it running. It is unfortunate and of the utmost concern that most people take better care of their automobiles than they do of their own bodies. People today are just too involved in extra time-consuming activities to participate in the normal mealtime of the pre-television era. Families no longer visit and chat amicably during meals. The air is now filled with the inane antics of forgettable television fare. The average child, for instance, spends one-third of his waking moments glassy-eyed before what has been aptly referred to many times as the "boob tube." This does not mean I do not appreciate the engineering ability and genius involved in transmitting sporting events, space efforts, political conventions, occasional good drama and comedy shows, etc. into my home; I am primarily concerned with our preoccupation with generally mundane and unproductive programming. A great majority of our citizens, both young and old, have become so addicted to television they rarely leave their sets except to go to work or school. This is not only very damaging to the eyes and optical system, it is a severe strain on the spine and related areas of the back. TV addiction also encourages a tendency to let things slide until tomorrow if only we can take an hour or two or three to watch the latest episodes of "Gunsmoke," "As The World Turns," "Medical Center" or "Dr. Marcus Welby" (or even a rerun of an episode seen earlier). As for physical exertion or exercise of any kind, the TV cultist has not the time nor the desire to "keep in shape." After all, with television, he can do it all vicariously.

It is often said: "You are what you eat." Truer words were never spoken, yet day after day people subsist on doughnuts and black coffee for breakfast; hamburger, french fries and cola for lunch; then rush home after a hard day's work to a frozen TV dinner. With this in mind, it is readily apparent that balanced meal planning as practiced so nutritionally by our grandparents is fast becoming a dying art. And so will we unless we start paying more attention to proper nutrition and adequate exercise and allow Mother Nature to once again influence our short earthly stay.

There is little doubt that our declining moral standards and fast pace of living are taking their toll. Although many people enjoy a longer life span now than ever before we also have the highest percentage of chronically ill in history. Now, what is the advantage of living longer if you become a victim of one of the incapacitating, degenerative diseases?

Is there a solution to the problem? I feel there is—and a relatively simple one at that. Most of us are aware that basic foods are good for us, e.g., raw, fresh vegetables, fruit and a variety of whole grains, both in cereal and bread form. Our biggest transgression has been in not taking enough time to properly prepare nutritious meals for ourselves and our families. Instead, we buy the already prepared quickie brand which takes three minutes to serve as compared to twenty minutes for the original product. What we too often fail to realize is that in order to give us this convenience, the manufacturer has had to sacrifice something beneficial. The basic nutrients are often destroyed by high heat or chemical processing needed to pre-condition the quickie food. Every time a food is heated part of the nutritive value is lost—what you are actually eating is a leftover warmed up again. Even more serious nutrient loss can occur with the chemical additives contained in so many of our food products today.

BASIC GUIDE TO GOOD NUTRITION

The cry of "What is there left for me to eat?" is a common one at this time. When our favorite foods are restricted, we are prone to feel nothing remains to eat and we will literally starve to death. Nothing is further from the truth. Your experiences in eating pleasures have just begun. Your waistline, vim and vigor and mental attitude will soon show you this is the way to go.

I have always refused to set up a daily menu for those who come to consult me for I feel it is impossible to outline a diet that will allow the individual to exercise his own ingenuity. The experience of selecting new foods and trying them out is a true pleasure for anyone concerned about the kind of food he takes into his body. In keeping with this reasoning, the basic dietary regimen which follows is a guideline which may be used by anyone who wishes to follow the Preventive Organic Medicine way of life. Since parts of it may be considered controversial, I will try to explain those which are most difficult to understand.

BASIC DIET

1. The following foods can not be eaten at any time: milk (pasteurized), ice cream, cream, pasteurized cheese, pork (including ham, bacon, sausage), canned meats, citrus fruit or citrus juice, alcohol in any form.

2. Any foods made with white sugar and white flour should be limited or cut out of the diet. This includes pastries, jams, jellies, most breads, prepared cereals, all soft drinks.

3. Foods should be prepared by means which preserve the most nutritional value: meats by broiling, baking, roasting—never by deep frying in oil; vegetables by steaming, waterless cooking. The more food eaten raw, the better.

4. Never mix a high carbohydrate food with a protein meal. As a general guideline: When eating meat, fish or eggs, do not eat fruit. Fruit and vegetables mix together well, as do vegetables and proteins. It is not advisable to eat meat more than three to five times weekly.

5. The less coffee or tea you consume the better off you are. Herb teas are encouraged.

6. Meals should be eaten slowly, with much attention given to chewing food thoroughly.

7. Regular elimination is a must. All steps should be taken to see that this is accomplished.

8. Regular exercise of at least two fifteen-minute periods each day should be observed.

One of the really controversial foods is milk. Very simply, it has been my experience that those who give up milk form less mucus, have less problems with constipation and in general are less congested. Pasteurized milk should be avoided at all costs, as the enzyme phosphatase, which is necessary for the body to utilize the calcium present in milk, is destroyed by the process of pasteurization. Thus, the calcium remains an insoluble mineral which could create problems of gallstones, urinary calculi, arthritic deposits, etc. The notion that milk is an excellent source of calcium is one of the greatest fallacies fostered by unknowing (we hope) officials and industry.

Milk also contains a pituitary growth-stimulating hormone which is necessary for the young but which can interfere with the endocrine system of the adult. Many endocrine disorders, including menopausal, thyroid and possibly even hypoglycemia, could be affected by an unusual stimulation of the pituitary.

Pork is, in my opinion, an unfit food for man. The unquestionable evidence of parasites which abound in the flesh of hogs should be a deterrent for most persons, but many have been lulled by the statement that thoroughly cooked pork does not contain active trichinae and is therefore safe. I recall an experiment performed with pork in which it was cooked at a temperature of 600 degrees Fahrenheit for over an hour. Now, this temperature is in excess of what the average housewife would consider using in cooking meat, yet when the pork was examined under an electronic microscope, more than twelve varieties of microscopic parasites were observed—alive and active. It is my belief that many of the problem cases of physical weakness not

responding to usually beneficial therapy treatment are
the result of a body infested with microscopic parasites.
There is much laboratory evidence to confirm this.

Almost all canned meats contain one or more
preservatives, particularly the nitrites. A nitrite is just
another name for what the veterans of World War I
and II called saltpeter. Such a substance has no place
in the diet of man.

Now for the problem restriction: No citrus. What a
thing to say in California, a state noted for its groves
and groves of fine citrus trees. I must, however, stand
on clinical evidence which has led me to the conclusion
that citrus fruit should be used only when it is eaten
completely alone—at least three hours before or after a
meal.

Many arthritics are aware that the use of citrus aggravates their condition and stay away from it because
of past experience. But why should such delectable,
God-given fruits be unsuitable for man's use? Perhaps
if man were still a vegetarian, citrus fruit would have
no inhibiting effect on his digestion and he could consume as much of it as he wished. However, the facts
are that man is inclined to eat large amounts of meat,
and the eating of citrus definitely inhibits the digestion
of any protein. Contrary to what many think, citrus is
not too acid but actually creates alkalinity within the
digestive tract, which prevents the proper digestion of
proteins and produces bloating, indigestion, gas, flatulence and, even more serious, the possibility of allergies. Remember that allergies are the end result of a
raw protein entering the blood stream.

I am fully aware that I am not going to stop everyone from eating citrus, but I wish to caution those who
are in ill health and who suffer from indigestion that

the use of citrus with your meal may very well be one factor in your problem.

It is also my opinion that rule number four of the Basic Diet should be carefully followed by anyone who wishes to preserve his gastrointestinal integrity. Those who are careful in the combinations of food they eat will find that eating becomes a pleasure and is followed by peace and contentment.

Since the other rules should be self-explanatory, I hope that the preceding outline will stimulate you to reorganize your eating habits in such a way that living becomes a joyful experience.

ENZYMES AND YOU

Recently I read a treatise by an esteemed nutritionist (at least he is accepted as such by scientific authorities) in which the author made statements so contrary to fact that my blood pressure rose and I picked up my pen to underline some of the more blatant misstatements. After reviewing his effort, I sat down and tried to rationalize calmly his purpose in writing such a book. The answer is quite obvious—certain special interest groups need such an authority to quote from when questions arise concerning the age-old controversy of live food versus dead food.

Some of the more offensive misrepresentations in the manuscript concerned the chemical structure of matter. I particularly object to the unsubstantiated theory that excessive temperature does not destroy enzymes or amino acids, but merely changes their structure. The author claims that when food is processed, the resultant chemical structure of the enzymes in the food has the same end result as the original unheated substance. To the uninitiated, this nutritionist might make sense, particularly if you remember some of your chemistry and the axioms and laws governing chemical changes.

It is fortunate, however, that dedicated and capable men such as Dr. Francis Pottenger conducted experiments with animals, using cooked food as sustenance for one group and raw food for another. Over a period of years, a clear unmistakable pattern emerged. Feeding an animal such as a cat pasteurized milk on a regular basis consistently produced arthritis; when raw milk was used, test animals maintained good health and agility.

Similar experiments and other documentation refute so-called scientific "facts" such as those given by the nutritionist in question when he states: "The faddist's claim that the destruction of the enzyme phosphatase in milk pasteurization destroys its food value is incorrect. It may be true that the enzyme is changed by the heat but its compound chemicals are still present so the food value of the milk is not altered."

Such reasoning must be compared to the ancient beliefs that the world is flat; that a large stone would fall more rapidly than a small stone; and other disreputable theories. The formula for such incorrect positions and assumptions lies in a steadfast adherence to self-induced theory without practical and time-consuming experiments designed to prove or disprove the validity of theoretical positions.

The enzyme phosphatase is necessary for the body to properly utilize the calcium and phosphorus in milk. In the absence of this enzyme the minerals are insoluble. For example, flour used by bakers to make commercial bread is always allowed to age a minimum of six months to guarantee consistency, a procedure assuring a minimum of enzymatic activity. Bakeries use this type of flour not with your good health in mind, but their investment. The lack of enzymatic action in commercial bread allows maximum retail exposure with a minimum return of stale or dated products to the manufacturer, hence greater profits. In this same vein, the nutrition-conscious housewife who insists on fresh whole grain flour is not always assured of an even, well-rounded loaf of bread because of the same natural enzymatic activity the commercial bakeries are so anxious to control. This is not written with an alibi in mind for any culinary misfortune you might have suffered in your kitchen but to explain and clarify that enzymatic action in flour (or any other food for that matter) has a great deal to do with what is served on your table.

Let us take a brief look at these miracles of nature called enzymes. Every one of your body's chemical reactions (which occur every second of your life) are directed and governed by enzymes. An enzyme is an organic substance, specific in function, which facilitates and accelerates chemical transformations and reactions. One particular enzyme will break down fats, another starch, another proteins; still others are concerned with the assembly of protein patterns for specific tissue repair and replacement. It is estimated there are over 80,000 enzyme systems in the body, each performing its own separate function.

Recent research indicates that lack or deficiency of certain enzyme systems is associated with, and may be the cause of, man's susceptibility to disease. This would explain the enigma of why one individual has heart disease while another member of his immediate family with similar eating habits and environmental factors suffers from arthritis. Enthusiastic researchers have stated: "A substance which will cure emphysema, arthritis, heart disease and tuberculosis sounds incredible, but a complete enzyme preparation has the potential of doing just that." The fact that the enzyme has not yet been harnessed in all its shapes and forms is all that remains to be conquered in man's quest for his answer to these problems.

Enzymes are protein in nature or composition, a fact in itself creating a vicious circle. An enzyme deficiency leads to lack of protein assimilation leading to an increased lack of enzymes resulting in even less protein assimilation. And around and around we go!

Common symptoms of an enzyme deficiency are bloating, flatulence, and poor digestion. Heartburn, an unfortunate aftermath of a heart condition, can also be due to lack of enzymes. The most commonly deficient enzyme of the digestive factors is hydrochloric acid. When buying a digestive aid, I recommend that a complete enzyme or complex of all the digestive factors be present (betaine hydrochloride, pancreatin, pepsin, papain, lipase, rennin, cellulase and bile salts). This formulation should provide a broad and adequate spectrum of digestants to properly digest your food. I should, however, point out that other factors (such as incompatibility of food) could create indigestion regardless of the digestive aids used. (More about this in Chapter III.)

YOUR LIVER AND YOUR HEALTH

The liver is often called the philosopher's stone, and rightly so. Throughout the years man has rubbed on it for the answers to some very weighty problems, particularly those pertaining to health, and often has come up with the right answers.

First, let us examine this organ. The liver is very aptly named—the liv-er. Without it, life is impossible. It is the largest gland in the body and the only organ which will regenerate itself if part of it is cut away. You can remove 25 percent of the liver and within a short period of time it will grow back to its original size and shape. Experimentally, a liver has been operated on to remove over twenty-five times the original weight of the entire liver and the organ still functioned normally. The liver will carry out its very important functions in the body if only 20 percent of it is active, without demonstrating any severe or noticeable symptoms.

The liver has many functions. The one with which we are most familiar is the secretion of bile. This fluid is stored in the gall bladder for release when needed. Bile is used in the body to digest fats and to aid in the absorption of fats, of fat-soluble vitamins (A, D, E, F, K), and of calcium. It also promotes peristalsis, therefore aiding in preventing constipation. Thus you can see that if this function of the liver is impaired, a myriad of functional disturbances could arise.

Food, after it has been absorbed into the blood stream through the intestinal wall, is put into the portal circulation and passed through the liver. Here is where much of the detoxification mechanism of the liver comes into play; also where nutrients are extracted from the blood stream to be stored in the liver for future use. These stored substances are utilized in times of physical stress and also for everyday activities.

The liver performs detoxification by combining toxic substances with other substances which are less toxic and which are, when combined, excreted—usually by the kidneys. Thus it can logically be concluded that for excellent liver function we must also have excellent kidney function. Conversely, we must have good liver function for good kidney function. Doctors have found that if either organ appears to be malfunctioning, it is wise to treat both for best results.

Another function of the liver which is not quite as well known is its relationship with the endocrine glands, particularly the sex glands. Malaise and loss of vigor are common symptoms of liver malfunction. Endocrinologists have found that the unfortunate male who has an excess of female hormones almost always has a liver problem. Insecticides and other poisons are all channeled through the liver in an attempt to detoxify them. A liver which is functioning well is, therefore, one of the best friends man can have in this day of almost universal exposure to insecticides.

Maintenance of proper levels of proteins in the blood is also dependent upon the liver. Since proteins are the building blocks of all the body cells and constantly need replacing, a malfunctioning liver could materially hasten the process of aging and also contribute to any degenerative-type disease. In fact, the Sloan-Kettering Institute for Cancer Research reports that test animals which were fed in such a way as to develop and maintain a healthy liver had almost 100 percent freedom from cancer as compared to other animals with as high as 33 percent susceptibility to various types of carcinoma. This should be food for thought for any individual who wishes to remain free from this scourge which now strikes one out of every three persons in this country.

Many more duties fall on the liver. In fact it has been estimated that for man to reproduce the function of the liver would take a chemical laboratory one story high, covering thirty square miles of ground. This organ carries a tremendous responsibility, yet few doctors are aware of the many symptoms which could be allayed by just restoring liver function to normal.

The obvious question arises: What causes liver malfunction and what can the average person do about it? I believe there are six basic reasons for poor liver function and a brief résumé makes them self-explanatory.

(1) Poisons which are cumulative in the system such as preservatives, insecticides and others. Even though the particular toxin does not accumulate in the liver—for example, sodium fluoride—the liver suffers because the pancreas and kidney function is not up to par.

(2) An improper diet ration—specifically low protein, high carbohydrate and high fat intake (particularly of saturated, hydrogenated fats). It is obvious that the low protein diet does not give the individual sufficient building materials for repairing and rebuilding. The high carbohydrate diet puts the individual on a high energy level right after eating, then subjects him to periods of virtual starvation because the pancreas has kicked out more insulin than was necessary to lower the blood sugar levels and the entire system suffers from a lack of vitality. This is why it is never wise to try and get a quick pickup from a candy bar or bottle of pop. Within a short time you are more tired than before eating or drinking the highly concentrated carbohydrate. On a high fat diet the liver must break down these substances into utilizable products. In the case of saturated fat, the entire process is useless because the end product is only harmful to the body anyway and imposes an additional burden upon the liver. In such instances, the liver often tries to store the fat in its own tissue, thus leaving less working area to be used for its many tasks.

(3) Poor quality nutrients are next on the list. The liver again tries desperately to make something useful

out of a substance that has been robbed of all its native nutrient values. On this list must come the refined white flour products, white sugar products, and imitation foods which appear to be, and even taste, similar to the original, but are without any vitamin, mineral or enzyme properties.

(4)   Probably the most common cause is overeating and overindulgence. The liver sucks up food like a sponge. Overeating and overindulgence create excess work and even bring about liver fatigue; then poisons are allowed into the blood stream without proper detoxification.

(5)   Although drugs are sometimes useful in emergencies, they inflict great strain on the liver. Allow me to explain why. Drugs are completely foreign and unnatural to the body. Their effectiveness lies in the fact that they create a reaction in the body which forces a particular organ to respond. Many times this response is that of a detoxification mechanism. The liver meanwhile is trying to eliminate the drug because it is a toxin. This is why a drug is effective for only a short period of time; the liver neutralizes its effect on the body. Incidentally, this is not true when organic substances are used to correct abnormal situations. In such cases the agent acts to fortify and aid the body.

(6)   Everyone is probably aware of the last factor—alcohol. Alcoholism is almost synonymous with cirrhosis of the liver. Alcohol acts much the same as a drug, with the liver finally giving up the battle and beginning to lose functional capacity.

For a few constructive hints on what you can do for your liver, I offer the following: avoid the aforementioned causes of liver disturbance; avoid constipation—the liver does double duty during such times; be sure your diet contains sufficient choline, inositol and lecithin; try to use a three-day juice fast once every thirty to sixty days. (See Chapter III for details on a complete liver-cleansing program.)

In 1964, a group of over forty doctors, each considered a specialist in the field of liver disorders, wrote a book devoted solely to liver problems. Their summary was particularly heartwarming. The regimen for patients suffering from liver disorder was as follows: bed rest, good food with adequate B vitamins and the withdrawal of any drug being used by the patient unless it was felt that it was necessary to preserve life. I only wish these recommendations would be followed more often.

THE GROUND RULES OF GOOD NUTRITION

Probably the two most frequently asked questions among those interested in the maintenance of natural health through good nutrition are: "What food combinations are compatible?" and "What combinations should a supplement contain in order to be beneficial?" The proper answers to such questions hinge on circumstances to a certain extent, but a few basic ground rules can be set which the average individual can easily follow every day, either at home or while eating out. These same rules can also govern choices of supplemental nutrition which you may feel are indicated for your needs.

The ground rules are simple. Once you have been exposed to them, meal planning or choice should be an interesting event rather than a confused, worrisome task. The following categories are not loaded with a lot of detail and explanation (although each could easily be the subject of a chapter by itself).

Category 1—ACID AND ALKALINE FOODS

These can be broadly categorized by saying that meat, fish, eggs, nuts, milk and cereals are acid-forming foods and vegetables and fruits are alkaline-forming. Care should be taken to include at least twice as much of the alkaline fruits and vegetables as of the acid-forming foods. It is important to note that the ultimate diet could become a simple routine by just following the above rule, but our modern foods confuse the issue because of changing chemistry during refinement.

Category 2—REFINED FOODS

You must avoid refined foods in every way possible and in this day and age that is a chore in itself. From roasted, toasted, double-dipped and shot-from-guns breakfast cereal to precooked, spoilage-retarded frozen dinners we are deluged with such processed, refined foods.

It is impossible to make a good, wholesome food out of a "dead" substance, and any food which has been precooked certainly cannot be called anything but "dead." Unfortunately, even the potatoes we now eat in many restaurants are partially cooked and then stored for easy preparation. This saves time and money but loses the most important ingredient—food value.

Many foods become harmful when they are no longer fresh. Oils are a good example of this; research has indicated that rancid oils are a possible suspect in certain malignancies. Yet we see oil in french fryers held over for periods of up to seven days with continuous use. This cannot help but be of concern; many authorities emphatically state that any oil should be heated up to the smoking stage only once, then discarded because rancidity immediately sets in.

We are a nation of refined carbohydrate eaters. Our cookies, doughnuts, pies, cakes, pastries, and other confections are a delight to the eye and a gross affront to the digestive tract. It is easy for students of civilization to distinguish refined carbohydrate lovers from those who concentrate on vegetables and fruits for their gustatory pleasures. It is also interesting to note the characteristic mental and physical actions of each group.

Sugar has been called the "curse of civilization." I would like to change that to: "refined sugar and refined foods are the curse of civilization." When we wake up to the fact that "foodless" foods are one of the greatest contributing factors in our constantly declining health, we will then reverse the downward trend and begin to build health again.

Since sugar consumption has risen every year to the point where the United States is the world's highest per capita consumer of refined sugar, I feel the following information should be made available in order that you might make your own decision as to whether you wish to continue your present rate of sugar consumption. The national average is almost 200 pounds per year for every man, woman and child in the United States.

Commercial sugar is made from cane sugar and sugar beets. Beet sugar is used much more extensively than cane sugar, therefore we will discuss the manufacture of refined white sugar from sugar beets. The first devitalization process is the removal of the top and neck of the beet. It is in this area that the heavy concentration of minerals lies; this must be removed in order that it does not interfere with the sugar crystallization. Then the juice is extracted by forcing water through the sliced beets. Since this extract is very dark in color, lime or carbon dioxide is added to precipitate some of the so-called impurities out of solution to clear it up. (Actually, these "impurities" contain nutrient value.) It is then centrifuged and separated into molasses and raw beet sugar.

The raw beet sugar is then thoroughly heated to destroy any life in the form of protein or enzymes which may still be present. Then animal albumin and bone charcoal are used as a filter to remove the dead protein in the mixture. Next the filtered material is thoroughly boiled again to separate the sugar from the syrup. The coup de grace is now administered—the sugar crystals are bleached with a strong bleaching agent.

Without a doubt, commercial sugar represents the ultimate extreme in food degeneration. After refining, it is almost a pure carbon, and when taken into the body carbonic acid is formed by the oxidation process of burning it up. Because all of the minerals have been removed, the body must call upon its mineral reserves to neutralize the carbonic acid which is a tissue toxin.

Refined sugar is a pure fuel without any food value. It is true that it will provide temporary and instant energy; but would you think of just adding gas to your car and never oil to the crankcase, not having it greased or not replacing tires when they are worn out? Gasoline can furnish fuel for your car to run on but it does not replace worn-out parts.

Refined sugar acts in the same way in the body. There are many sources of natural sugar which will supply our needs for fuel but which are integrally combined with vitamins and minerals necessary for maintenance and repair processes in the body.

Did you know that soda pop contains at least seven teaspoons of refined sugar per bottle? Most candy is almost completely refined sugar with perhaps some artificial flavors. These artificial flavors, along with artificial sweeteners such as saccharin, are derived from coal-tar derivatives. Such coal-tar derivatives have been named as a definite causative factor in cancer. And, in many European countries, such sweeteners are restricted to prescription only.

You can make up your own mind, but I know where I am going to obtain my fuel from now on!

Category 3—OVEREATING

This is without a doubt one of the most common errors in all nutrition. In this land of plenty we never consider the fact that nature intended us to eat only when we are hungry, not when the clock tells us that it is time to eat. I know that many will criticize me for this statement because it will upset their routine or schedule. On the other hand, many have demonstrated the health value of eating only when hungry and have found this to be an excellent way of regulating their weight without being conscious of every bit of food taken into their mouths.

In order to establish such an eating pattern I would recommend that you go on my liver-cleansing program, then gradually begin drinking a variety of vegetable and fruit juices and work into solid foods. In this way your body will have a chance to direct your path and you will not be dependent upon that conditioned reflex which the three-meals-a-day program actually is.

When eating a meal, chew your food thoroughly and try not to mix a protein and a carbohydrate in the same meal. There has been much controversy about food combinations and it is true that certain individuals are capable of eating almost anything and not suffering any ill effects. But it is a good rule of thumb to observe the above suggestion for optimum digestion. If you eat a protein meal containing meat, eggs, etc., use vegetables with it, but no fruit. On the other hand, when eating fruit you may mix vegetables with it, but no high protein food.

Category 4—RELAX WHILE EATING

In this hurry-scurry world we often have so much on our minds that the act of eating is purely mechanical, while the brain is operating at a furious pace trying to figure how the bank account can possibly balance this month, or what to do about Johnny's bad teeth. Our Latin neighbors, who take a siesta after eating, and people in the countries where dining is a multi-course performance with great care given to what many of us consider minor details, all have a built-in advantage for food utilization and assimilation. The very act of recognizing the food we eat and considering it in the mind creates gastric secretions which enhance digestion. It is far better to skip a meal than to rush through it.

Category 5—EXERCISE

Exercise is to health what oil is to the squeaking wheel. Without it, degeneration soon sets in and the "wear and tear" types of disorders begin. There is no greater fallacy than "I am too tired to exercise," or "I don't have time to exercise." A vigorous fifteen minutes, morning and night, will create energy that the average person didn't know he was capable of. There are so many good devices available and so many simple exercises that can be done in almost any situation, that any excuse for not exercising is simply invalid. More and more doctors are beginning to recognize that exercise is the very best recovery medicine available for almost any disorder.

The foregoing ground rules are practical and easy to

follow. Should you decide to observe them you will obviate many visits to your doctor; and when you do decide to consult with your nutritionist, you will save him much valuable time in educating you in principles.

DIGESTION

"I CAN'T BELIEVE I ATE THE WHOLE THING"

One of the most important factors in nutrition is good digestion. Digestion begins in the mouth. Many people are totally unaware that in many instances, upset stomachs and intolerance to certain foods could be avoided by proper mastication of food. When food is taken into the mouth and the process of masticating or chewing it begins, several important functions in other parts of the body are set in motion to receive the food after it is swallowed.

The enzymes and digestive juices which are so necessary for proper digestion and utilization of food are stimulated by reflex action by the type of food which is being masticated. Hydrochloric acid from the stomach, pancreatin from the pancreas, pepsin from the stomach, bile salts from the liver—all are dependent in part on getting a message through reflex channels from the mouth. The salivary glands in the mouth produce the enzyme ptyalin which acts upon starches immediately, beginning their breakdown to assimilable products for human nutrition.

Horace Fletcher (1849-1919), American nutritionist who attributed his own health to the thorough mastication of his food, wrote and lectured widely on nutrition, popularizing his ideas until "Fletcherism" and "to Fletcherize" became part of the American language. After many years of illness and poor health during an active and varied business life, he turned his attention to research in the field of human nutrition (from 1895) and in his later years continued to outclass many young athletes in endurance tests. The major factor contributing to his extreme good health involved a comparatively simple formula—chew all your food until it is swallowed without volition; that is, without conscious effort to swallow. He also recommended abstinence from extremes, such as hot or cold liquids or heavily spiced foods. "Always allow the senses of the mouth to tell you what will be comfortable and acceptable to your stomach," is as good a statement as any to sum up his philosophy and way of life.

I heartily concur with this man. How many of us are addicted to gobbling our food without regard to what will happen after it reaches the stomach? How many of us gulp down hot drinks and ice water because we cannot stand them in the mouth? If we cannot tolerate such things in the mouth, just think of the poor esophagus and stomach! No wonder reflexes are improperly triggered; no wonder indigestion occurs.

Another excellent advantage in using Fletcherism is that a person never overeats. Appetite does not shut off like a current of electricity, but gradually wanes just like the setting sun. If we eat hurriedly, we not only risk poor digestion but also overeating, because the reflex center that tells us that our hunger is sated never has a chance to bring the message.

In summary: (1) Take your time eating. (2) Chew your food thoroughly. (3) Never abuse your stomach with extremes such as hot or cold. (4) Remember, if it is unpleasant in your mouth, it will certainly be unpleasant in the rest of the digestive tract.

After food has been mixed with saliva and is passed on to the stomach, it is almost immediately besieged by several secretions which are necessary for proper digestion to occur. The stomach itself secretes hydrochloric acid and pepsin. Bile from the liver and pancreatin from the pancreas complete the major secretions. Contrary to popular opinion, hydrochloric acid is not the most important of these secretions although it should be emphasized that we cannot do without any of them and have normal digestion.

The most important secretion is pancreatin which, with its enzymes, digests proteins, fats and starches. Hydrochloric acid and pepsin act in a secondary manner to back up the pancreatic enzyme function. Bile, the secretion from the liver which is stored in the gall bladder, acts as an emulsifying factor for fats. Bile is produced at a slow, constant rate by the liver, then stored in the gall bladder where, upon stimulus, it is dumped into the stomach. This is one of the reasons why people who have had the gall bladder removed surgically have difficulty digesting many foods, particularly the fats. The bile is secreted at a rate too slow to cope with any large amount of fat in such circumstances.

Inadequate secretion of these digestive factors brings about many symptoms including discomfort, diarrhea, constipation, flatulence, headaches, anemia, hypoproteinemia, belching and many others. It is a known fact that the production of these secretions begins to decline at about the age of forty. At this time, it is important to eat foods which stimulate and act as helpful agents for the proper secretion of gastric juices. Beets and beet tops, preferably raw or lightly cooked, are particularly recommended as a food in these cases.

For those who have undergone surgery and thus lost function of one or more of these secretions, it is advisable to see your doctor for advice on replacement in tablet form of the active factors that promote good digestion.

Now we take the food into the small intestine. Here we begin the assimilation process—in other words, absorption of the elements which have been broken down by previous digestive processes into simple factors which the body can use.

The intestinal villi, the tiny root-like protrusions into the intestine from its wall, literally suck up the digested food and pass it into the portal vein. The obstruction of these villi with undigested food can be a definite cause of malnutrition and/or nutritional deficiencies. The main reason for such an obstruction is undigested food—primarily due to lack of digestive secretions—and constipation.

Constipation can many times be controlled merely by increasing the intake of fluids and bulk in the diet. In addition, certain foods such as flaxseed and many herbs are effective in this condition. Some diets can cause constipation. The low sodium diet, for example, contributes to constipation because sodium is an essential mineral for normal tonicity of the intestinal wall. Without sodium, the walls become atonic and peristalsis is slowed down. If you must restrict sodium intake, then eat a lot of raw vegetables.

After our food has passed into our portal vein, it is routed to the liver. The liver acts further to process the food and serves as a "storage tank" to regulate its release into the blood stream. Thus, the liver is the main organ of assimilation or metabolism of nutrients after they are absorbed through the intestinal wall. It therefore has a great role in our resistance to disease, in maintaining a proper blood sugar level and in dictating our appetite or craving for certain foods.

The residue which is left after the nutritive value has

been absorbed from the food then passes to the large intestine or colon, as it is often called. The colon is divided into three parts: the ascending, transverse and descending colon. It is larger in diameter than the small intestine but shorter in length. The undigested and undigestible matter accumulates in the colon until it is evacuated.

It is easy to see that the colon is an ideal area for toxic buildup. With constipation as prevalent as it is, it becomes a definite factor in many symptoms which are common today: headaches, indigestion, nervousness, insomnia, etc. Nature has provided friendly acid bacteria in the large intestine to prevent the multiplication of toxic bacteria. However, it has been the unfortunate experience of many, particularly those who have been given large doses of antibiotics, to find that these bacteria are no longer present to protect them. In all of these instances, the possibility of constipation is greatly increased as is the possibility of absorption of toxins through the bowel wall and back into the system.

These friendly organisms can be reintroduced by using a retention enema containing the acidophilus bacillus or by the simple expedient of taking various preparations which contain them, by mouth. Yogurt has long been used for this purpose.

As mentioned before, peristalsis is necessary to properly empty the bowel. Exercise, particularly walking, plays a large part here, and should be a part of the daily routine of anyone interested in good health.

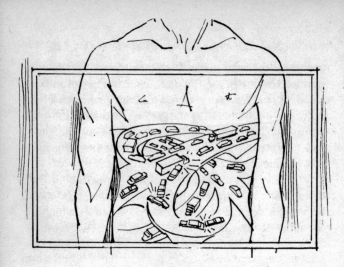

Chapter III

THE CONGESTED FREEWAY

ALTHOUGH THE average layman knows more about his physical body today than ever before, many are still unaware of the intricacies of the gastrointestinal tract. They know of the small intestine, the large intestine and other general areas, but are not conscious of the fact that the gastrointestinal tract extends some thirty feet in length and is a convoluted, tortuous path which can have many dead-end side roads and single-lane expressways only to bottleneck itself back down to a single lane.

Man was originally intended to partake of many and varied raw fruits and vegetables, whole grains and fibrous meats. The very nature of this fare kept his intestinal tract free of debris because the roughage and fibrous content was adequate to stimulate normal elimination. One other advantage that man had many years ago was the absence of plentiful and convenient transportation. As a result, he sometimes walked several miles a day in the performance of his duties. This walking was a boon to his intestinal tract because it stimulated peristalsis, that wave-like motion which moves the contents of the tract along. (Note: He may have had a built-in heart attack preventive in this measure, also. Most cardiologists now recommend that all their heart attack patients begin a walking program as soon as possible.)

Today the exact opposite is the rule. We are transported by mechanized means to our destination, be it one block or 100 miles away. This transportation doesn't jolt or vibrate our bodies; in fact, auto manufacturers praise the "smooth as silk" ride of their particular make or model. We sit in plush chairs which do not necessitate changes of posture, for they are contoured to fit the body. Our food is mainly pre-prepared, overcooked and de-fibered, so that we have a homogenous mixture requiring very little mastication before being swallowed. The habit pattern is then set, and foods which should be chewed are hastily swallowed.

The vast number of patients seeking medical help for gastrointestinal problems such as diverticulitis, colitis and ulcers could be greatly decreased with proper attention to our food and its proper preparation—which includes adequate chewing. We spoke about the dead-end side roads in the intestinal tract. These are the diverticula, small pouches or pockets opening off from the main intestinal tube, which often fill with feces and set up irritation, inflammation and even abcesses. It stands to reason that it is not an easy task to wash these pockets out at will, so we must try to correct the cause of the diverticulum, or pouch, rather than give only symptomatic relief. Once such a pocket has developed, it will be a constant source of irritation; and since bland foods tend to be less irritating, the sufferer will just keep on living with his condition and deteriorating physically because of an inadequate diet.

There is an answer. Many doctors of Preventive Organic Medicine are aware of the relationship of low glandular activity to colitis, for example. The body is not capable of restoring and repairing tissue when glandular activity is at a low ebb. There are several means of restoring such function, including eating a high quality protein diet, balancing the mineral elements which are necessary for glandular function, supplying glandular extracts for specific glands and using vitamin E as a hormone precursor. And for goodness' sake, let us not forget exercise!

Recently, I read an article by an eminent doctor who had done research on the relationship between thyroid and iodine. It was his contention that iodine in an organic state, such as is found in sea food, has never created an excess of iodine in the body, regardless of how high the intake was. In sea food, which includes kelp, we have an excellent high-quality protein and also an excellent source of mineral elements which are often lacking in glandular malfunction. An abundance of such foods in your menu will assure your glandular system of the building blocks it needs for proper function.

Many are unaware that there are glandular extracts available which do not make claims for hormone activity but are supplied as specific protein factors for glandular rejuvenation and restoration. Normally, these are available only from a doctor, but they are very much in keeping with the theory of organic medicine. Vitamin E has played so large a part in heart disorders that many overlook its very important function as a hormone precursor or trigger.

All the above-mentioned factors will help you to keep your digestive tract healthy. Allopathic medicine has pretty much replaced the Sippy diet with chemical preparations designed to coat the intestinal tract. Common sense will tell you that this constant coating does not heal, but only subdues the symptoms temporarily. Give your body a chance to tone up, and know the peace and happiness that come from the inner glow of natural health.

THE NEED FOR DETOXIFICATION

You are feeling OK. As far as you know, there is nothing wrong with your health. Why, then, do you need to detoxify?

If you are of the opinion you need to detoxify only when you are sick or exposed to poisons, you are entirely wrong. In fact, what makes most people sick is the loss of the ability to detoxify their own wastes of metabolism—wastes which are easily disposed of by a healthy person but inflict an ever-increasing load upon the body machinery of one whose detoxifying system is somewhat less than efficient.

The body's ability to detoxify its normal metabolic wastes is the best way of judging a person's general health. It is, in effect, our main bulwark against the ravages of the polluted atmosphere in which we find ourselves. How, then, can building up the detoxification mechanisms help us to combat this inescapable stress?

The detoxification systems of the body can be likened to the flue on a furnace. The body is constantly producing heat as a result of the combustion of fuel we

consume. If the diet is high in protein and only unrefined fats, sugars and starches are consumed, this
natural food burns up and leaves little ash to be
handled by the detoxification mechanisms. But when
natural efficiency is dampened by the introduction of
almost pure chemicals such as are contained in highly
processed sugars and starches, the result is like closing
off the flue of a furnace. The combustion smolders,
toxins accumulate and a vicious, continuing cycle is
formed.

Dr. Alexis Carrel (1873-1944), French surgeon and
biologist, first developed methods for suturing blood
vessels and transplantation of organs, then proved that
a heart fed in a test tube could be kept beating for
many years. The recipient of the 1912 Nobel prize for
physiology and medicine had this to say about toxins
resulting from his celebrated test conducted with isolated live tissues:

"To a piece of living tissue in a test tube we have to
add an amount of fluid which is 2,000 times its volume
in order to prevent its being poisoned in a few days in
its own wastes."

If the tissues of the human body were detoxified in a
similar manner, it would require about 50,000 gallons
of fluid to do the work. How this task is accomplished
with only six or seven quarts of blood is the phenomenon of life called detoxification. To a great extent, its
efficient function depends upon how well your body is
fed.

In another landmark experiment, Dr. Sydney Ringer
(1835-1910), English physician known for his work in
clinical medicine and physiological research on the influence of organic salts on the circulation and heartbeat
(and after whom the famous Ringer's Solution is
named), showed how concentrations of minerals fed a

heart muscle could be either physiological or toxic, according to the proportions of each present in the feeding solution. When concentrations of potassium (an esential mineral) were increased, the rate of contraction became weaker and slower until the heart muscle finally ceased beating. When calcium (another essential mineral) was increased in concentration, the reverse situation occurred.

The muscle pulsated at a faster rate with the contractions becoming quicker and stronger until, finally, the heart stopped beating in a state of contraction known as "calcium rigor." Dr. Ringer proved that although both calcium and potassium are essential to health, they must be in ionic equilibrium and in proper proportions. The thyroid and adrenal glands are instrumental in regulating this delicate balance in the body. One of the effects of stress—including environmental stress—is putting abnormal burdens upon these glands (and the pituitary gland) in maintaining the internal environment.

There is little doubt that every essential nutrient—and many functional nutrients—are concerned with the process of detoxification simply because they affect the body as a whole. However, some nutrients are much more concerned with the process than others. The vitamins which enter the methyl-donor and -receptor reactions are particularly important. These reactions are necessary for conversion of fats and oils to energy forms, amino acids to proteins and other intermediate chain reactions in metabolism. Vitamin B-6 forms the hub of the wheel of this group, surrounded by choline, niacinamide (B-3) and vitamin B-12.

Highly important in the detoxification processes are the minerals potassium and calcium. Potassium, in particular, is required in steady intake as the body (kidneys) has little or no means of controlling its excretion from the blood stream, even when the cells are severely deficient. Potassium seems to have special powers in promoting healing; a deficiency of this important mineral appears to be the cause of lowered mechanisms.

The intestinal tract does not enter directly into the detoxification process. Its environment must be considered independent of the body chemistry itself. Imagine it as a long hollow tube running down through the center of the body, actually an "external" surface similar to the outer skin. The intestinal environment can be secondarily important in toxic conditions, because unless the digestion and absorption are normal the bloodstream will not be properly fed, regardless of the quality of the diet.

Food not completely digested before entering the intestinal tract can be a source of fermentation, putrefaction and rancidity (starches, proteins and fats, respectively). In maintaining the intestinal environment, digestive enzymes are particularly important as a preventive measure.

Deleterious by-products of faulty digestion can be precipitated by the use of absorbents, the most natural of which is pectin in its colloidal form. In fact, this is the basis for the saying, "An apple a day keeps the doctor away."

As we have pointed out, detoxification is a normal process; its efficiency is an index of health. Good nutrition is necessary for optimum detoxification. Conversely, poor nutrition holds it back. A diet free of purified, highly concentrated foods such as white flour and sugar is the first step in assisting the detoxification processes. Supplementing the diet with special vitamins, minerals and proteins can also assist the detoxification processes. It is the bringing of all ends toward the middle that is of primary importance. We must remember that the whole of human health is derived not from the sum of its apparent parts but is equal to much that is yet to be explained in human consciousness and is possible only through faith and trust in a Supreme Healer.

THE DETOXIFICATION PROCESS

I have long advocated that the most important factor in any disease condition is to first detoxify the body, then treat whatever symptoms remain. When patients are informed about the many benefits of detoxification, they soon realize that the so-called average diet of today is insufficient and woefully lacking in proper nutrition and life-giving substances. It soon becomes apparent that dis-ease is not always or even necessarily due to a variety of the latest "bug" in vogue at the moment (as we commonly explain symptoms of discomfort and ill health today), but can be related to a toxic condition within our own bodies. More physical and mental problems than not are created or caused by simply eating the wrong foods and lack of physical exertion.

As a result of extensive research and much practical application, I have developed what has proven to be a particularly effective combination approach to a short-term detoxification program. It is comparatively simple and easy to follow, particularly so because the onset requires only three days. Of course, there are some who will not benefit from this program because of pathological situations which could cause severe reactions. However, as a general rule, if you are not under the care of a medical practitioner for an acute or chronic disorder which requires continuous medication, and do not have ulcers or other acute disorders of the intestinal tract, it will prove beneficial for you to follow these simple suggestions:

Start with a Liquid Fast of three days' duration as outlined below:

1st day: Drink 1½ cups fresh lemon juice mixed with sufficient honey to make palatable in two quarts of water. Also, separately, drink the juice of sufficient raw beet tops and roots to make two fluid ounces.

2nd day: Repeat same lemon, honey and water mixture but increase beet juice to four fluid ounces.

3rd day: Repeat lemon, honey and water mixture but increase beet juice to six fluid ounces.

Remember, drink the lemon, honey and water mixture throughout each day of the fast. The recommended daily intake of beet juice may be divided as desired, but the indicated ounces for each day *must* be consumed for optimum results.

Beginning with the day following your fast, taper off gently, adding other liquids as desired; delete citrus juice of any kind from your diet. Abstain from eating any refined white sugar or white flour products, drinking pasteurized milk or consuming any other pasteurized dairy products. It is recommended that meat, preferably chicken or veal, be eaten no more than four times per week; pork and processed meats should never be considered.

The general feeling of well-being and renewed life which follows this detoxification program will encourage you to regularly utilize it at least once every four to six weeks. Such rejuvenation of your liver will allow this vital organ to function at peak efficiency and provide you with the basis for continued good health and vitality.

Although the foregoing is the basic detoxification

program, there are some common variations depending on the requirements of each individual case.

For the patient with chronic constipation, the addition of one quarter teaspoon of Epsom salts to the Liquid Fast each morning and night is recommended.

If the patient has an extreme aversion to lemons or an allergy, substitute carrot juice diluted as follows: three parts carrot juice to one part water totaling two and one half quarts of solution to be consumed as needed throughout the day. Apple juice or grape juice similarly diluted is also acceptable.

A word of caution: It is extremely important that the specified quantity of liquid is taken into the system each day; the success of your fast depends on strict adherence to the rules without exceptions. If by any chance nausea is produced or the beet juice should prove distasteful to the patient, it is permissible to dilute the beet juice with a small amount of water, celery or apple juice or a combination of all three. For the quickest and longest-lasting results, however, undiluted beet juice provides the optimum results in the shortest period of time.

Continue to abstain from the eating of any meat or heavy protein for a period of from five to ten days. The more raw food eaten during this period, the greater the cleansing action and more complete the detoxification process.

I can not stress too strongly the importance of regularly cleansing the body, particularly the liver. It is of the utmost importance to the maintenance of good health and long life. The detoxification program outlined here can be very easily implemented without losing any time from your daily activities and without loss of energy or stamina. After starting this program many patients report feeling refreshed by it, and having more

energy on the third day of their fast than when they
started. This is not true one hundred per cent of the
time, of course, but a feeling of euphoria and well-
being is not uncommon during short fasts.

THE TOTAL FAST

There are numerous other methods often used to
cleanse the body. The Total Fast, in which the individual drinks only water, has been a time-honored and
proven remedy for many ills. My only objection to this
is the imposition on the individual's strength and the
objectionable breath odors, etc., which accompany
lengthy water fasts. If the patient wishes to put himself
under a doctor's care, prolong the fast beyond three
days and is fully aware of the ensuing drain on his energy, it can be a fantastic method of losing undesirable
weight and ridding the body of accumulated toxins. If
this method is undertaken, I highly recommend spring
or well water be used as I am convinced distilled water
tends to leach minerals out of the system. It is my
opinion that the mineral balance in the body can be
more essential than vitamins or other considerations, so
I repeat: Do not use distilled water in any detoxification program you decide to try!

Variations of the water method are many. I have
used aqueous chlorophyll in water for two to four days
for many conditions with excellent results, particularly
in stomach and intestinal disorders. A multiple herb tea
or a single herb has also been used satisfactorily (sas-
safrass, flaxseed, ginseng, golden seal and many others
all have cleansing properties) and can be used for
short periods of time to fit into everyday living patterns. For best results, fasts undertaken without a doctor's supervision should remain short (three days or
less) and used more often. Detoxification crises can

flare up which are just as acute and damaging as any disease-caused crisis; competent professional advice should always be sought if the problem being treated persists.

THE MONO DIET

Advocates of the Mono Diet are becoming more and more numerous although this approach also has many variations. Basically, the idea is to utilize a basic food which causes very little strain on the body yet provides sufficient and adequate nutrition. The primary benefit of this approach is the elimination of improper food combinations. Most American diets create extreme difficulties for the body in its effort to properly use the food we do eat. This condition is completely avoided in the Mono Diet as the body utilizes fully that which is consumed. A great variety of foods can be used in this fast (rice, avocados, papaya, watermelon, to name a few), but to my knowledge the only food sufficient to sustain life indefinitely is the raw potato. (By sustaining life, I refer to a life without deficiency disease, a worthy goal for us all.)

For those afraid of the hunger pangs that a fast usually creates, the Mono Diet for a short period of time might prove the most advantageous to try. Another program quite similar to the Mono Diet is the Juice Fast; only one kind of juice is consumed for a period of several days. Both certainly have a great deal of merit and can be utilized with success under proper conditions and supervision.

Although we have barely scratched the surface of the many and various types of detoxification programs available, the basic outline for relief and treatment of sickness and disease and preventive procedures to safeguard good health in the future have been presented.

Many times bowel function is overactive at first, then tends to slow down as the body cleanses itself. It is advisable to maintain open bowels at all times but an over-concern with this function is not necessary or desirable. As the body normalizes, the bowel will usually regulate itself. If the problem should persist, I repeat, the reader should seek professional help and advice.

An interesting sidelight to the subject of detoxification is the fact that many of the truly great personalities of all times were aware and cognizant of the tremendous benefits of periodic fasting. Many religious sects today still practice this ancient and proven method of healing and preventive medicine.

This writer's own personal experience on the lecture platform has taught him to fast for at least twelve hours before appearing in public as a speaker or master of ceremonies. I find my mental processes are much clearer, there is better tone to the body and my physical reactions are much sharper. Fast—and ye shall age slower and live longer! You have nothing to lose but a little unwanted weight and good health to gain if you detoxify—so why not give it a try?

THE CREATIVE RESTORATION DIET

This diet is designed for you—a health program for modern living between fasts. A great deal of study and practical clinical experience has resulted in this concise and precise program. Your participation can only be as effective as your application of the rules. As anything worth doing is worth doing well, why not accept this restoration program as a real challenge? Put it to work for you for a mere thirty days of your life; in return, you will benefit by improved health and good living, the greatest wealth of all.

INCOMPATIBLE HABITS

Certain habits are incompatible with your search for health. You cannot build with one hand while tearing down with the other and expect to fashion a monument. The following are incompatible with good health:
1. Consumption of alcohol. This has been proven scientifically to destroy brain as well as liver cells.
2. Smoking. So much evidence has been presented that we need not elaborate.
3. Over-consumption of coffee and tea. Both of these contain habit-forming drugs and are deleterious to the central nervous system. You may substitute herb teas (available in health food stores) or use vegetable or cereal beverages.

UNDERSTANDING THE CREATIVE RESTORATION DIET

This is a recommended method of eating foods to induce you to automatically improve your diet. *It must be understood*, not just blindly followed. You must learn to lead your own way. Unlike the dull, restricted menu-type diet which requires discipline to enforce, this educational approach can be interesting. It encourages a greater, rather than lesser, variety of foods, thus both taste and appetite are more likely to be satisfied. There is also a great satisfaction in being able to select foods by reason of good judgment and common sense, rather than by the usual hit-or-miss method.

Therefore please read the following information carefully. If you understand why you are asked to follow certain rules and guidelines, it will be much easier to give your cooperation. It merely takes plain, common sense and a wisp of willpower. Your conscience should become your guide.

Since this diet consists primarily of vegetables, meat, fish, poultry and fruit, it is high in minerals, especially potassium, an essential mineral of prime importance in the body chemistry. Because it is high in fermented foods, which are rich in lactic acid, it encourages a favorable intestinal environment. It is intended to eliminate a high proportion of so-called "empty calorie" foods, so it should have an excellent normalizing influence on your weight.

Naturally, not all of the foods which one should not eat can be mentioned. In this regard, only the major classifications are given, listing a few categories only. The guidelines for food combinations to be avoided are few and easy to follow. Emphasis is placed upon the positive what-to-eat nature of dieting. It is a diet you can believe in because it is founded on truth, rather than fancy or statistics.

SIX BASIC GUIDELINES (OR RULES) TO FOLLOW ARE LISTED AT THE END OF THIS CHAPTER: THEY SHOULD BE LEARNED AND PRACTICED UNTIL THEY BECOME MATTERS OF HABIT.

GENERAL PRINCIPLES OF THE CREATIVE RESTORATION DIET

I—REGARDING WHITE FLOUR AND WHITE SUGAR PRODUCTS

Not only are white flour and sugar products devoid of their naturally occurring vitamins and minerals, but the less desirable calories are concentrated until they become little more than pure starch and carbohydrate. How is this abuse of nature's stores brought about?

In the case of white flour, shelf life is the main reason. All commercial white flour is processed so that it can be stored for long periods of time. To make this possible, most of the "life" is removed from the whole wheat berries. Since the oil is removed, it cannot turn rancid (although wheat germ oil is very important to health). Everything subject to oxidation has been removed. If it were not so, spoilage would be rapid, often within a period of a day or two.

White sugar is refined for another reason. In its liquid form as cane juice, it would ferment rapidly and would require refrigeration from cane field to user. Obviously, this would not serve commercial purposes. Granulated sugar does. But the attendant loss of vitamins and minerals, plus the intensive concentration of purified carbohydrate, make a mixture too rich for your metabolism to handle efficiently (like the carburetor on your car when too much gas is mixed with the air).

An important feature of the Creative Restoration Diet is to eat maximum quantities of live foods and eliminate those foods which are purified concentrated substances; WHITE FLOUR PRODUCTS AND WHITE SUGAR PRODUCTS ARE NOT LIVE FOODS SO MUST BE ELIMINATED!

It is comparatively simple to eliminate much white sugar from the diet simply by not eating candy, pastries and so forth. However, many find it difficult to eliminate all white flour products such as bread and paste foods (macaroni, spaghetti, pizza and the like). The elimination of white flour products is essential, however, if the fullest benefits are to be obtained from the Creative Restoration Diet.

II—REGARDING THE USE OF UNCOOKED FOODS

Let us look at your diet from the aspect of how much of it consists of uncooked or raw foods. Many people go days on end with no more raw food than a smattering of lettuce or an occasional glass of fruit juice. The remainder of their diet is completely cooked.

THE EATING OF FRESH, RAW FOOD DAILY SHOULD NEVER BE LEFT TO CHANCE. A vegetable juicer (not liquifier) is ideal for this purpose and lends itself to a wide variety of raw foods prepared as liquids which may be drunk. Those fortunate enough to be in an area where fresh carrot juice is available should never miss the opportunity of feasting on this exceptionally healthful raw food drink. If these facilities are not available, two outstanding all-season foods are recommended as follows:

(1) TOMATOES AND TOMATO JUICE
(2) RAW CABBAGE

Canned tomatoes, without preservatives added, are on the list of acceptable foods. Tomatoes are one of the few vegetables which lend themselves well to the canning process. In fact, because tomatoes are canned at the height of their natural perfection, the food value can be higher than the hot-house varieties sold in off-seasons. The same applies to tomato juice, both rich sources of potassium and vitamins A, B, and C.

Salads made with raw cabbage instead of lettuce can be one of the greatest taste surprises you have ever had. Cabbage in raw form is one of our richest sources of essential vitamins and minerals. It stores as well, if not better, than any other raw food, keeping its nutrients through many winter months beneath its protective wrapper in the leaves. The value of eating cabbage as a winter-needed raw food was extolled by the Roman emperor, Cato, who gave a discourse on its many merits as a health-building food. His wisdom has now been well substantiated by scientific proof of its nutritional ingredients.

WHETHER CARROT JUICE (OR OTHER FRESH VEGETABLE JUICE), RAW CABBAGE OR TO-MATOES, IT IS INDISPENSABLE TO THE SUCCESS OF THIS DIET THAT A HIGH QUAL-ITY RAW FOOD BE INCLUDED IN THE DIET DAILY!

III—Use of Meat Products in the Diet

Meats, such as veal, beef, liver and so forth, are good sources of protein, as are milk, cheese and dairy products in general. However, even though the protein intake may be adequate insofar as quantity is concern-ed, quality is an even more important point to consider. Incomplete protein leaves pieces of the "building block" mechanism unfinished, and, like a jigsaw puzzle with pieces missing, the whole protein picture suffers. This is good reason to supplement the diet with a specially processed protein product to assure an ade-quate amino acid supply and balance.

Also in regard to protein ingestion, its liquification into amino acids is essential to its utilization. This is called the process of digestion. If digestion fails to liq-uify the meat (protein), spoilage can occur in the in-testinal tract, a process called putrefaction. This is good reason to supplement the diet with an appropriate digestive enzyme product.

Contrary to some opinions, the grinding of meat into small particles, e.g., hamburger, does not increase its digestibility. Nor does the thorough chewing of meat. No protein digestion occurs in the mouth. Meat need only be chewed to the extent that it may be easily swal-lowed. Meat-eating animals tear their foods and have no molar teeth for chewing.

On the other hand, the grinding of meat can have deleterious effects. Ground meat spoils rapidly at room temperature; whole meat does not. In fact, aging of whole meat can make it more nutritious by a sort of "pre-digestion" which occurs in the process.

It is postulated that nucleic acids are released when meat is ground, coming out with the meat juices and apparently making spoilage very fast. Similar action may occur when ground meat is introduced into the intestinal tract. Here the temperature is ideal for rapid spoilage. This is particularly applicable if there is insufficient hydrochloric acid in the stomach, as HCl acts as an intestinal antiseptic to inhibit fermentation and putrefaction which might otherwise occur. Here, again, a proper digestive aid containing hydrochloric acid sources may be used to distinct advantage.

Note: Preserved meats, such as weiners and sausages, do not have as much tendency to putrefaction, since they contain anti-putrefactive chemicals (usually nitrites or nitrates) which work both inside and outside the body to produce this effect. HOWEVER, FOR THE SAME REASON, PRESERVED MEATS ARE NOT DESIRABLE FROM A NUTRITIONAL VIEWPOINT.

IV—USE OF SUGAR AND PROTEIN COMBINATIONS

One of the little known deleterious effects of refined sugar is its effect on protein digestion. Sugar, depending upon its relative concentration, inhibits or retards the action of proteolytic (protein digesting) enzymes. Therefore, sweet foods (such as desserts high in sugar) should not be eaten at the same time as animal source (protein) foods. As an example, beans, such as navy beans, are an excellent source of protein. In Mexico, beans serve as a major constituent of the diet, much as potatoes do here. The Mexican diet calls for unsweetened beans. In Mexico, beans are not considered a gas-forming food, but in this country, where they are served with molasses as sweeteners, and sugars, they are well-known as a gas-forming food. This illustrates the deleterious effect of sugars on protein digestion.

Too many Americans are accustomed to finishing off a good protein meal (steak or other meat) with sweet desserts (apple pie, for example). Desserts or foods high in sugar, even natural sugars, are best eaten several hours after meals. All sweets should be eaten on an empty stomach for proper nutrition.

There are many sugar-protein combinations which may be easily avoided if one is on the alert; chocolate milk and sugar-cured hams are outstanding examples. The fact that most foods contain some protein must be taken into consideration; a small amount of sugar does little harm, of course. It is the *concentration* of the sugar which is the important factor, its deleterious effects being proportional to the quantity present.

V—USE OF FERMENTED FOODS IN THE DIET

One of the first methods discovered for the preservation of foods was by fermentation. Such foods as pickles, sauerkraut, buttermilk, yogurt, cheese, and cottage cheese came into being as a result. All of these foods, in their natural form, have a long history of use by the human race and are highly acceptable as dietary items.

Because the fermentative process acts to produce lactic acid, this natural acid is common to these foods. Lactic acid in this natural form is well-known to have a "sweetening" effect in the intestinal tract, acting as we know today to promote the growth of beneficial intestinal bacteria, thus improving the intestinal environment.

Two foods are outstanding in the fermented foods

class: (1) buttermilk, and (2) sauerkraut and sauer-kraut juice. Both are readily available and are rich sources of lactic acid. Buttermilk is preferred, of course, because of its higher protein content. But those who do not care for buttermilk may use sauerkraut as a source of lactic acid (eaten raw as packed in the container; kept in the refrigerator in a closed jar to prevent the spread of odor).

VI—REGARDING THE USE OF COMMON SALT IN THE DIET

People who eat as much salt as they like may excrete nine times as much potassium, an essential mineral, as those on salt-restricted diets. Actually, Americans frequently consume 20 to 25 times as much salt as estimated sodium requirements allow. If this is not counter-balanced with increased potassium intake, such as is found in vegetable juices, a borderline potassium deficiency state can be induced by such salt excesses. It is always wise to use salt as sparingly as reasonable seasoning will allow.

A new modified herb salt is available that automatically decreases the sodium intake of salt added to foods by 50 percent, without loss of salty flavor or taste. In addition the product increases by 50 percent the potassium intake from this source. This modified salt is not a salt substitute, since it does contain salt, but it is an excellent way to reduce salt intake for persons not on prescribed low-sodium diets, such as persons on reducing programs and those whose salt restriction seems to be otherwise logical.

ADDITIONAL COMMENTS AND SUGGESTIONS

"Don't eat between meals" may be poor advice. There is nothing against snacking, when good wholesome food is used. Tests on animals and humans have shown that there is less weight gain and better health when they are given free access to food than when the usual practice of regulated feeding intervals is followed, such as the "three square meals a day" plan. Excellent snack foods are: eggs, celery, carrots, nuts, fruits, tomato juice, grape juice, figs, dates, etc., as well as protein tablets.

Raw potatoes, especially if eaten immediately before retiring, have an excellent laxative effect, no doubt due to the high raw potassium content. The effect can be enhanced by taking about an ounce of the following combination: ⅓ cider vinegar, ⅓ honey, ⅓ blackstrap molasses, prepared in advance. This is then diluted with water to taste. It makes an excellent non-fat salad dressing as well, adding a sweet-sour flavor which is acceptable to most people.

SUGGESTIONS FOR SUPPLEMENTATION WHILE ON THE CREATIVE RESTORATION DIET

In general, the diet itself is abundant in natural vitamins and minerals. However, its overall nutritional pattern can be augmented by the use of those supplemental formulae which may be particularly indicated for your individual nutritional problems.

OVERALL PICTURE OF THE CREATIVE RESTORATION DIET

In order to help you obtain a better idea of the recommended diet, examples of desirable and undesirable foods are listed here. (Of course, not all foods can be shown, but study of the examples given will suffice to show the type of indications necessary for best results.)

DESIRABLE FOODS:

1. ALL GARDEN VEGETABLES (fresh, frozen, canned, in order of preference, respectively) such as: asparagus, beans, peas, carrots, potatoes, broccoli, sweet potatoes, yams, rutabagas, tomatoes, chard, lettuce, celery, cabbage, etc.

2. MEAT DISHES AND SOUPS such as: steaks, roasts, stews, vegetable soup, potato soup, boiled dinners, etc.

3. FERMENTED FOODS such as: buttermilk, yogurt, cottage cheese, other natural cheeses, sauerkraut, and pickles (unsweetened).

4. FRUITS, FRUIT JUICES AND VEGETABLE JUICES such as: tomato juice, grape juice, pears, avocados, apples, etc.

UNDESIRABLE FOODS:

1. (a) COMMERCIALLY PROCESSED FLOUR PRODUCTS such as: bread, biscuits, rolls, cookies, crackers, doughnuts, spaghetti, macaroni, pizza, pie crusts, dumplings.

(b) COMMERCIALLY PROCESSED WHITE SUGAR PRODUCTS such as: soda pop, candy, pie, cake, etc.

2. GROUND OR PROCESSED MEATS such as: ground meat, hamburger, meat loaf, weiners, sausage, chili, hash, luncheon meats.

3. SUGAR-PROTEIN COMBINATIONS such as: baked beans, ice cream, chocolate milk, desserts with meals, sugar-cured ham, malts and milk shakes, sugar in coffee with meals.

BASIC RULES OF THE CREATIVE RESTORATION DIET

1. Eat no food products prepared from commercially processed white flour or white sugar.

2. Drink at least one glass of tomato juice and eat one serving of raw cabbage daily.

3. Avoid the use of ground or processed meat.

4. Never combine high concentrations of sugar with proteins at one time or at the same meal.

5. Include some form of fermented food in the diet daily.

6. Eat high proportions of natural, raw and unprocessed foods.

NOTE: The above dietary recommendations are for general nutritional purposes only and are not to be considered substitutes for any specific nutritional counsel or advice of the doctor concerning specific situations depending upon evaluation of the individual involved. Certain persons considered experts may disagree with one or more of the above statements or recommendations.

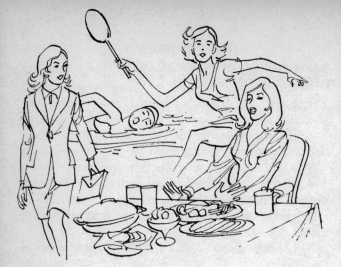

Chapter IV

RESISTING POOR HEALTH NATURALLY

THE AGE-OLD refrain, "I catch everything that comes along," is a common complaint today. On the other hand, there is the individual who never seems to be affected by anything; doesn't "catch cold" or get the "flu," and any wound heals rapidly without attention. The person who seemingly is subject to every infection finds it difficult to understand this paradox and often complains in a manner similar to the obese individual who knows that he doesn't "eat enough to keep a bird alive."

There is a simple and logical explanation for this which, though largely unknown, can be of invaluable assistance to everyone who understands the mechanism involved. A few years ago, the *Reader's Digest* published an excellent article entitled "The Useless Gland That Guards Our Health." The gland involved is the thymus, a tiny lump of tissue located behind the breastbone. For many years, this gland was considered useless after the first few years of life. In fact, its true function is as a form of "mastermind" which regulates the intricate immunity system to protect us against infectious diseases. Research has indicated that when the thymus is removed from animals they lose their ability to cope with small inoculations of infectious bacteria which normally would have been no problem.

An interesting and intriguing addendum to this is that more recent research indicates the appendix, tonsils and adenoids also may have a part to play in the immunological response. In the patient who is deficient in gamma-globulin, for instance, tests have shown the thymus to be defective; in almost all cases the tonsils had been removed or were severely underdeveloped.

Now we come to an even more interesting facet of this whole story: How does the thymus, and possibly other glands, affect the body's response to invading bacteria? In the case of the thymus, we now know it is the originating source for lymphocytes, the small, white blood cells responsible for resistance to infections. Although they comprise only about 1 percent of the total white blood cells, the absence or reduction of lymphocytes is directly proportionate to the degree of body resistance.

These tiny lymphocytes eventually leave the thymus, spreading to the spleen and lymph nodes where they rapidly grow and multiply. The lymph nodes are a part of a network (in all probability hundreds of miles long) which comprises the lymphatic system. This system is so minute, only the most powerful and up-to-date microscopes can enlarge it sufficiently to be examined by the human eye. The system is so complex and fragile that many of the lymph ducts collapse under even the most delicate probing.

DRAINAGE SYSTEM

Exhaustive and dedicated research and practical application have determined that this lymphatic network acts as a drainage system for the cells, and to carry nutrients and impurities back to the blood stream. In order to nourish cells, blood capillaries constantly leak minerals, fats, vitamins, proteins and sugars into the extracellular fluid. These nutrients are then absorbed by the cell and the wastes expelled. It is reasonable to consider that much of this nutrient matter is not utilized by the cell and here is where the lymphatic channels come in. Without such a network, we would literally begin to bleed to death in a short time. Precise and informed calculations lend credence to the theory that half of the blood protein is lost from our veins every twenty-four hours. If the lymphatic system did not retrieve and resupply this protein, disaster would soon occur.

EXERCISE IMPORTANT

The lymph system does not have a pump to propel the fluids along the lymphatic ducts, an omission which provides an excellent reason for exercising both isometrically and isotonically. It appears that lymph fluid is propelled mainly by the activity of the body: breathing, walking or any other muscular activity. Such activity moves the lymph to the thoracic duct where it finally empties into the blood stream.

Other functions of the lymph also include the most elaborate filtration system ever created, to filter out invading bacteria. An innate intelligence directs this filtering-out process, resulting in harmful material accumulating in bean-shaped masses of tissue known as lymph nodes. These nodes are far too numerous to even contemplate; if one is overloaded, there is usually another equally capable of doing the job. It is interesting to note how these nodes work. All of us have seen the enlarged lymph node in the armpit or groin after cutting a finger or foot; when this happens, it indicates the local lymph nodes in the area of injury were not able to handle the problem. Since the armpit and groin are areas of lymph node concentration, they were called on to help overcome the infection.

Even more intricate are the other functions of the lymph system, one of which is the measured release of fats into the blood stream at a rate which does not alter the chemical balance of the system. This is necessary because a high blood fat concentration can lead to destruction of red blood cells.

Since lymphocytes mature and grow in the lymphatic system, a mechanism is set up whereby an enormous increase occurs when the body is under stress of invading bacteria. Hormones are then thought to be carried in the lymphatic system to various other areas where they trigger functions important to daily life.

Such a vast and involved network is certainly well worth our time and effort to enhance its function. We can readily see why isometric exercise is important to the bedridden patient in order that the lymphatic channels remain active, maintain circulation of life-giving nutrients and filter out dangerous substances. It has long been popular to use certain herbs to help cleanse the lymphatic nodes as a precaution should the body be put under stress (common varieties are sarsaparilla, lobelia and golden seal). Most of us are familiar with other protective measures to be taken in time of infection; should we not give some thought to our natural rivers of defense?

COMMON SENSE AND SLEEP

Rip Van Winkle's record sleeping session must stand forever as the envy of all insomniacs. The subject of sleep is one that has been studied intensively by physiologists for years and still very little is known about it.

Perhaps this is what makes the interpretation of dreams so fascinating.

Let us investigate sleep and see what a bit of common sense will tell us.

You will never see a hungry baby go peacefully to sleep, so it stands to reason that an adult will not fall peacefully into the arms of Morpheus if his body is starved of essential nutrients from within.

Of these nutrients, three are outstandingly important:

1. The Lullaby Mineral: calcium (which should be in ionizable form).

2. The Kaleidoscope Vitamin: vitamin B-6 (a daily intake of at least 50 mg is necessary).

3. The Balance Wheel Mineral: potassium (most effective in the chloride form).

Now the question to be answered is this: Will taking a food supplement containing these nutrients in proper amounts make you fall to sleep easily? Not necessarily.

Here is a story to illustrate the point. McCollum, a famous early American nutritional scientist, was lecturing to a group of newspaper editors on the pacifying effects of magnesium (best source—magnesium oxide), when one of the more skeptical participants challenged: "Do you mean to tell me that if I take magnesium, I'll have a pleasant, amiable disposition?" To which McCollum replied, "No, I doubt that magnesium alone would do that, but putting your present outlook on life aside, it would be pretty hard to improve your disposition without it." So as far as sleep is concerned, all that nutrition can do is remove one of its obstacles.

Theda Bara brought glamour to the early movies by being photographed on a leopard skin. Can you think of a more enticing way to pose? Yet there is more to this idea of sleeping on pelts than nostalgic remembrances of past publicity stunts. Pelt therapy has now become widely accepted as a preventive treatment for bedsores in hospitals. At first, only sheepskin pelts were used. Now synthetic fibers have appeared on the scene.

Bedsores develop in areas where the flesh is kept compressed for periods of time. Pelt therapy has considerably relieved the stress. Why?

If you press down on the thick natural fur of a sheepskin, you realize that it would be literally impossible to stop the circulation of air under your hand. The thick fur allows the circulation of air under the affected part, making pelt therapy effective in the control of bedsores.

What has this to do with sleeping?

In European health spas, it is a common practice to use air bathing as relaxation therapy. The belief is that the air flowing over the surface of the body sends multiple sensations to the brain which, in turn, produce a natural sedative effect. It does not take much prodding of the imagination to understand that a similar effect can be obtained by sleeping on a sheepskin pelt. This is far superior to linen bedding, cotton or wool which actually do little more than provide warmth. I have talked to many persons who have tried this procedure for inducing restful sleep. All are pleased with the results.

Raw onion has long been known as a sleep-inducing food (although its social aspects are not beneficial). The same applies to potato-garlic soup, a most soothing food for the insomniac to eat before retiring. But perhaps the most famous home remedy of all is a glass of warm, raw milk before retiring. This has been a time-honored recommendation made by doctors to mothers of restless children. This is more than just an "old wives' tale."

Raw milk causes a rapid rise in blood calcium levels (calcium is the sedative mineral). This can be demonstrated by a simple urine test. I am not suggesting that this test be given any practical application, but cite it merely to show that often some of grandma's favorite remedies were based upon keen observation which later scientific investigations proved correct.

I think the best advice to give to an insomniac is that he rests almost as well without deep sleep as with it, providing he does not wear himself out worrying. The nitty-gritty of the whole thing is that most of us do not know when we are actually asleep. Many people do their best thinking in a semi-sleeping state.

The all-important thing is to retire with an "I-don't-care" attitude and allow nature to do the rest. Many people have been amazed at the amount of rest (and sleep, though they will not admit it) which is obtained when they stop worrying and simply go to bed to rest. If you want to be frank, it is pretty hard to go even one night without any sleep at all—even for insomniacs.

NATURE WON'T WAIT

It has long been the innermost desire of so-called civilized man to thwart nature, be it in the realm of synthetic foods or in any of a number of other areas which are highly questionable. It was brought to my attention recently that a study by some leading medical researchers indicated an alarming correlation between mental retardation, epilepsy and permanent brain damage and a common practice in our hospital delivery rooms: the procedure of holding back delivery of an infant until the attending physician arrives on the scene.

Such a procedure may have a certain amount of appeal for the fearful young mother or the nervous father, or the society matron who would not think of applying even a Band-Aid without the permission of her physician. It is unfortunate that we no longer look upon childbirth as a completely normal and natural function of the female of the species. I have observed many young women who abhorred the thought of the unpleasant task of childbirth; on the other hand, I have spoken with many who had taken a course in natural childbirth and who reported that giving birth was one of the great moments in their life.

Regardless of my personal feelings on the matter, I believe that the following facts should be considered before we allow convenience to dictate to nature.

Dr. William F. Windle, a leading authority on the physiology of the newborn, and Dr. Charles Carter, an authority on retardation, recently completed a study which demonstrated that the practice of holding back delivery creates an oxygen deficiency in the baby's brain at an extremely critical time. Such an oxygen deficiency could result in irreversible brain damage, which may be cerebral palsy, mental retardation or epilepsy. If the work of the two doctors is accurate (and every indication points to such an assumption), then 60,000 cases of mental retardation, 30,000 cases of epilepsy and 7,500 cases of cerebral palsy can be directly traced to such hospital procedures. It was also noted that these figures do not take into consideration the development of epilepsy in later life, an occurrence which can often be directly or indirectly traced to injury at birth.

The physiology is simple, insofar as the oxygen deficiency is concerned. Until the moment of birth, the unborn baby receives oxygen from the mother through the umbilical cord and the placenta. At the moment of birth, the infant's lungs take over. The well-being of the child depends on the successful transition from one source of oxygen to another, in a precisely-timed and well-regulated sequence. If the birth is delayed at this crucial transitional stage, even for a few minutes, serious brain damage may result.

According to Dr. Windle, recipient of the $10,000 Albert Lasker Award for Basic Medical Research for his studies of the human embryo, holding back the infant is something most doctors do not want to talk about. Everyone knows it takes place, but little has been written about it. It is an unpublicized procedure, and there is reluctance to come to grips with it. Up until 1965, when Dr. Carter published a paper on the hold-back maneuver as an obstetric danger, many hospitals still observed regulations that delivery should not take place without a physician present.

Such regulations should be scrutinized carefully. Every hospital has an obstetric facility with nurses who are assigned to duty there. Some of these obstetrical nurses have observed more births than the average doctor and are well capable of assisting in a normal delivery. Why should nature be held in abeyance while a doctor gets another few hours of sleep? Many possibilities immediately come to mind, but since this can only be conjecture, it is better for expectant mothers to have a good talk with their doctor or consider natural childbirth as an alternative.

It is interesting that Dr. Windle cites widespread ignorance among members of the medical profession for the shocking number of brain-damaged infants. Poor preparation of doctors in medical schools, particularly in the areas of embryology and physiology of the fetus, and the fact that there just are not enough doctors to go around too often lead the medical profession to try to schedule what should be an event of nature. It is unthinkable that anyone would knowingly take the risk of harming a newborn, but the unfortunate fact is that information concerning the danger of the hold-back practice is not necessarily common knowledge in the medical profession.

The trend of the American public to no longer accept medical errors without redress is a healthy one, as it enables conscientious individuals such as Dr. Windle and Dr. Carter to publish their work and also to speak out in public on some practices within their own profession which are not in the public interest.

Your doctor is one of the best friends you can have in an emergency, but you most certainly have the right to know his viewpoint on matters which concern your health and the health of your children. Practices which are contrary to nature should be avoided.

HELLO, FATTY!

The subject of hyperinsulinism (also known as hypoglycemia) has been of much concern recently as more and more becomes known about this syndrome. Unfortunately, many people are still confused on the subject and a simplified discussion may prove helpful. In particular, it may be enlightening to the overweight person who has been frustrated for years trying to reduce, but still has a problem.

There are, of course, those people who are overweight simply because they eat double portions every time they come near food. They make no bones about it, they just have a gargantuan appetite. The sad thing about this is that if they were not suffering from hyperinsulinism before, they will probably soon develop it. Hyperinsulinism is an excessive production of insulin brought about by the stimulus of concentrated sugars originally, and eventually by almost any food which is eaten by the individual because of his craving for a food high in sugar or carbohydrates. This excess secretion of insulin immediately acts on the sugar in the blood stream to burn it up as energy or store it in the cells as fat. Since more insulin is produced than is necessary to burn up the amount of sugar present, a condition of low blood sugar (hypoglycemia) results. Since a normal blood sugar level is necessary for all normal functions of the body (particularly those of the brain), the innate intelligence of the body sends out a high priority message that it needs more food. Needless to say, this only perpetuates the vicious cycle, i.e.: high carbohydrate food creates excess insulin which depletes the blood sugar rapidly which creates a hypoglycemic condition which immediately triggers an alarm system within the body, demanding more high carbohydrate food.

With the exception of the strain on the pancreas, the condition would not be so serious if the sugar were completely burned up; but the sad fact is that the greater portion is stored as fat. The stored fat is never tapped as a source of energy by the individual because of his dietary habits, which usually include an over-abundance of carbohydrate food and a minimum of protein. This excess fat then goes on to create problems of importance in the body; circulatory, glandular, etc. When almost 75 percent of our population, in my opinion, is afflicted with liver malfunction, you can be assured that the fat person undoubtedly suffers from this problem. This makes it much more difficult for his doctor to rehabilitate any bodily function because of the prime importance of the liver in normal body activity.

A malfunctioning liver is a detriment which must be considered thoroughly by the treating physician. Although a high protein diet is of paramount importance to control and overcome this hypoglycemic condition, the sluggish liver cannot properly handle proteins and convert them into sugars which will dribble out slowly into the blood stream and maintain a normal blood sugar. A physician I know who has probably treated more hyperinsulinism cases than fifty average doctors combined has recognized this weakness and compensates by trying to cleanse the body, first by using a Mono Diet (the patient is allowed only one food in addition to the supplements and cleansing preparations used). As liver function slowly returns, additional foods are included with the emphasis on low carbohydrate and high protein foods. Most people need a complete enzyme digestive aid during this phase because of the importance of as nearly perfect digestion as possible. It must also be emphasized that the hypoglycemic patient is similar to an alcoholic; the first concentrated sugar ingested can bring the whole cycle into existence again.

The title of this section was used in order to obtain

the overweight person's attention. Research has demonstrated that 90 percent of the fat people tested suffer from chronic hyperinsulinism (hypoglycemia). The fierce desire for soft drinks, candy, pie etc., which is experienced by these individuals is not a sign of inadequate willpower; it is an uncontrollable innate command to procure food which will temporarily raise the blood sugar and do it fast. After the subsequent overflow of insulin, the storing of the sugars as fat becomes a side effect and complication of the basic condition and eventually makes it worse.

We all know the individual who seems to be able to adjust food intake to energy output and thus never gains weight. This is particularly true in the animal kingdom with one important exception: when you introduce starches and carbohydrate foods to an animal, he will get fat and lazy the same as we humans. This should be adequate cause and reason to reevaluate your diet immediately. Dr. Weston Price and countless other able researchers in the field of the relationship of diet to health have reported that until refined flour and sugar were introduced, most chronic health problems known to civilized man were nonexistent.

To make crystal clear the reason for the production of an excess amount of insulin we should recognize that the human physiology is not set up to handle concentrated sugars. When such concentrated sugars are ingested, they bypass the normal channels of digestion and are rapidly absorbed into the bloodstream. Since such a concentration of sugar could bring about a coma such as the diabetic is subject to and can produce death in a short time, an emergency signal is sent to the pancreas to send up a big supply of insulin to combat this excess sugar in the bloodstream. In the diabetic, the pancreas cannot respond because of lack of function and insulin must be administered by other means or the glandular function restored by natural means. However, in the normally functioning pancreas, a big load of insulin is produced as a protective mechanism and dumped into the bloodstream. The insulin makes short work of the excess sugar, but in so doing usually depletes even the normal blood sugar. The brain, which uses the sugar in the blood as its chief fuel, now begins to send out ever stronger signals that it needs some *right now*. The intense desire for food is initiated and because of our plentiful supply of artificially concentrated sugar products (such as soft drinks, pastries, etc.) the cycle begins all over again.

It would be an ideal situation for the hypoglycemic to live where he did not have such concentrated carbohydrates at hand. Unfortunately, this is not easily possible and the knowledge of what they do is necessary to motivate people to avoid them. In order to adequately treat this serious condition, the following should be observed: 1. Find a physician who is cognizant of the facts of hyperinsulinism. (Many physicians are still prescribing sweetened juices and candy bars to overcome hypoglycemia.) 2. Have a 5-hour glucose tolerance test to determine the severity of your condition. 3. Stay away from all refined carbohydrates and synthetically sweetened foods. 4. Follow the advice of your physician as to the cleansing program needed in your case and carefully adhere to the diet recommended even though it may become monotonous. 5. Use foods which are high in protein and eat small amounts of these foods 5 to 6 times a day. 6. Use a natural, organic food supplement furnishing a broad-spectrum vitamin-mineral complex. 7. It is usually advisable to use a *complete* digestive enzyme complex with your meals.

By following these suggestions, it is possible to reorient your entire body to normal. The excess fat will amazingly seem to melt away; hypoglycemic headaches will disappear; hyperirritability and inability to cope with everyday problems will be relieved; and periods of depression and lack of energy will no longer be present.

FLUORIDATION AND YOUR HEALTH

I feel it is imperative that certain facts on fluoridation of water be established for the information of the public. In so doing, we will remove all doubts from the minds of any who have questions as to my position or the factual evidence supplying the reason for my taking such a stand.

Sodium fluoride is a poison! Sodium fluoride is the type of fluoride proposed to be added to the water supply of all of California and, if successful there, to other states in the union. The proponents of fluoridation will immediately answer that many waters are naturally fluoridated to a far greater extent than they propose. The important fact that the natural fluoride is in the form of calcium fluoride is not even mentioned. The basic chemical difference is that calcium fluoride is comparatively insoluble or, to put it more plainly, is extremely difficult to dissolve, while sodium fluoride is readily soluble and as such will enter the tissues of the body quite easily—calcium fluoride cannot. Sodium fluoride is classified by law as a poison in the same category as arsenic and cyanide.

Sodium fluoride is a poison in the dilution of 1 part per million. The proponents of fluoridation, when confronted with the fact that sodium fluoride is a poison, return with the statement that the dosage of 1 ppm* is

*ppm - parts per million.

insignificant and nontoxic. The studies, scientific or otherwise, on which they base these claims express opinions by someone either pro-fluoridation or nonexistent. At this time there has been no prolonged study of the safety factor of adding sodium fluoride to the water supply of man. On the other hand, scientific evidence, well-documented and carefully controlled, would indicate that sodium fluoride, even in minute concentrations, is a toxic element when introduced into the human system. I might bring up at this time a seemingly contradictory position of the Food and Drug Administration: they have banned the use of sodium fluoride in prenatal vitamin formulae, but say nothing about the addition to drinking water. Is it not just as inadvisable to add it to our universal, natural water supply?

The concentration of 1 ppm of sodium fluoride in water is sufficient to cause cellular degeneration and/or allergies. A film narrated by Jonathan Forman, M.D., clearly demonstrates the enzyme-inhibiting action of sodium fluoride on the cellular structure of animals. Normal cellular activity is shown, with the growth and division of cells. Then sodium fluoride, in a concentration identical to that proposed as safe, is added. Before your very eyes you see the cellular activity slow down— cells become smaller, less cell division takes place and finally the cell dies. It is accepted practice for all drugs to be tested on animals and if they demonstrate untoward effects they are not licensed for sale. Here we have clear-cut evidence of the toxicity of sodium fluoride and yet proponents tell us it is harmless.

As you have probably noted, all three of the aforementioned points are regarding the toxicity of sodium fluoride. This is one of the most important considerations that must be clarified before any other aspect of this proposal is discussed. As a doctor, it is my moral obligation to present to you factual evidence which would clearly indicate that the addition of sodium fluoride to the water supply would and does create physiological problems of grave importance. The following is offered as evidence.

It is admitted by proponents of fluoridation that concentrations of 4 to 5 ppm could have a detrimental effect on the human physiology. By advocating a 1 ppm concentration in the water, the proponents completely overlook the possibility of other fluoride ingestion. Tea is particularly high in fluoride; many of the foods we eat contain fluoride and as we will point out later, the atmosphere we breathe may well be loaded with it. I recall a report from a little town in Montana called Garrison, in which the farmers asked for and received $123,000 in damages from a phosphate plant which emitted fumes causing their animals to lose appetite, give less milk, produce malformed calves and develop bad teeth. The toxic element in the fumes was fluoride, according to the newspaper story.

Let me quote from the *Missoulian*, a local Montana newspaper: "In Garrison, the landscape and its community of life are dying—slowly succumbing to the fluoride threat." A further quote will show the frustrating logic of the law: "More important to the rancher plaintiffs than any compensation for past damages was the requested permanent injunction terminating the defendant's (the phosphate plant) operation at Garrison, for here was their only guarantee against continuing damage." The injunction thus far has been refused, so the agony and bickering continue—as does the destruction.

This particular story includes pictures of several excellent examples of fluoride toxicity—pictures of the fluoride-damaged lower jaw of a cow; another picture of a cow hobbling on its knees suffering from exostosis, a bone disease produced by fluoride poisoning; another picture of the damage to the evergreen trees by fluoride fumes. Such evidence is amazing to the person not familiar with aspects of fluoridation other than those propounded by fluoridation advocates. It behooves us to be aware of the following facts which are in direct contradiction to the statements made by fluoridationists.

The addition of sodium fluoride to the water does not stop or prevent decay. It has been demonstrated that it delays the eruption of permanent teeth so that a statistician could present figures which would indicate that there is less tooth decay in children who drink fluoridated water than in those who drink non-fluoridated water. Remember: figures don't lie, but liars figure. If a child has fewer teeth in his mouth, it is rather obvious that he will have less decay, right? United States Public Health records clearly indicate this dentition delay. It is the opinion of many experts that by age twenty the decay rate of fluoridated teeth is as high or higher than that of the non-fluoridated.

The addition of 1 ppm always causes some fluorosis or mottling of the teeth. It has been the contention of profluoridationists that if 10 percent or less of the population had a certain degree of mottling, it would be considered negligible and without significance. Yet the criteria for fluoride poisoning is the detection of mottled teeth. This is by no means the only symptom of fluorosis, but it is the easiest to detect. Let us discuss for a moment the actual physiology of mottling of the teeth. A tooth is formed of many types of tissue of which enamel is the hardest and acts as the exterior covering for protection. This enamel is formed by cells called ameloblasts—fluoride tends to poison these ameloblasts.

The same situation is present in the formation of bone. The latest tactic of fluoridationists has been to say that the addition of fluoride in water would also help our older people who suffer from osteoporosis because more calcium is retained by the body when fluoride is ingested. They reason that this calcium is then utilized by bone tissue to strengthen it. This is not always so! It is true that osteosclerosis, which is an increased calcium content of the bone, has been produced by fluorides. It is also true that the amount of fluoride required to do this would be the equivalent of about 50 to 60 quarts of water per day at a concentration of 1 ppm. Does this make sense?

The paramount fact which is overlooked in this assumption of benefit is that osteosclerosis is a disease condition in itself. It is many times associated with anemia because the extra calcium begins to infringe on the marrow space of the bone where red blood cells are formed. The American Medical Association has issued a warning to this effect but it has been ignored by fluoridationists.

The fluoride ingested by humans can be detected in large quantities in soft tissue structures such as the kidneys, the parotid glands, skin, arteries and others. There is an apparent association between such concentrations and various diseases such as kidney disease and arteriosclerosis. Such correlation should make any scientist step back and say: "Let us find the facts, do some research on this before we bring about another thalidomide scandal." Sweden, a country noted for its scientific advances, has rejected fluoridation completely. Should we not inquire as to the reasons why?

I have attempted to give you some of the major dangers in fluoridating our water supply. May I urge those of you who are interested in more detail to write the National Health Federation, P. O. Box 688, Monrovia, California, for their book on the subject entitled *Fluoridation*. It is a most complete treatise written by experts, in a language which the lay person can easily follow.

WHY SOME NEED SUPPLEMENTS MORE THAN OTHERS

If you live in a hilly area you may need vitamins more than if you live on the plains. Nebraska, a flat area, for example, has a rich, deep topsoil—fifty feet deep in some places—and the terrain is covered with a thick covering of buffalo grass. The dense top covering keeps down the growth of trees because they cannot take root in this environment. Hilly areas, on the other hand, erode easily and the topsoil is thin because it is washed away. This makes good fodder for trees and their presence makes a deceptive impression of the fertility of the soil.

Such an area is found around Wilkes-Barre, Pennsylvania. What do this city and Nebraska have to compare? A report of the United States Department of Agriculture titled *Human Nutrition* gives us an answer. Nebraska has the lowest death rate in the nation; Wilkes-Barre has one of the highest.

It seems evident that well-intentioned persons in both areas, following recommendations for a well-balanced diet, would be consuming varying qualities of 'foods—vitamins, minerals, proteins and the like. When comparisons are made on a national level, using the lowest and highest death rates of these areas, here is what we find:

If Nebraska's death rate is used: 138,365 less persons would have died.

If Wilkes-Barre's rate is used: 410,489 more persons would have died.

This is a difference of 272,124 lives.

That is quite an impressive figure, but when death rates for this country and other countries of the world are compared, the quality of the diet takes on even greater significance. The same USDA report shows a list of death rates for 20 countries. The United States ranks 18th, the Netherlands lowest. This is also a lowland country of rich agricultural produce. Apparently the dikes were well worth the effort.

So when somebody says, "I eat a well-balanced diet and don't need to take vitamins," ask them, "Where do you live and where were you raised?" If the answer isn't Nebraska or the Netherlands, it would seem that taking vitamins would be a wise procedure—and even in these plush areas taking them would not do any harm.

Another reason why some people's need to take vitamins is greater than others' is what scientists call "biologic variability." This means that an individual's nutritional requirements are related to his own constitution. Some persons may need so many more vitamins and other nutrients to stay healthy that deficiencies can crop up in spite of a well-balanced diet which would be adequate for most people.

An interesting demonstration of this principle occurred with the release of prisoners of war after World War II. Some showed signs of severe deficiencies while others, who had eaten the same food, were affected only by the loss of weight. Little is known about the upper limits of nutritional requirements, but the evi-

dence on hand is strongly in favor of a high intake so
that a sufficiency for all persons is assured.

Another constitutional condition which affects significant segments of the population is called "lactose
intolerance." Lactose is the sugar found in milk (milk
sugar). It can not be absorbed into the bloodstream
until it is converted to glucose or galactose by an enzyme named lactase. This enzyme is lacking in those
who are intolerant to drinking milk. In these people,
the lactose is acted upon by bacteria in the intestine
(which are always present) to cause the production of
gas and the accompanying discomfort of diarrhea and
abdominal distention.

A USDA bulletin reports that 19 percent of white
persons are so affected, 74 percent of blacks and 95
percent of Orientals. It is no wonder that milk is often
refused when given in free lunches to children in ghetto
areas where there may be a predominant percentage of
blacks. Since milk is a prime dietary source of calcium—invariably recommended in "well-balanced" diets—it becomes obvious that lactose intolerant persons
need to obtain this essential mineral by supplementing
their diets with a compatible calcium source.

The prevention of nutritional anemia is another condition calling for more supplementation of the diet by
some persons than by others. The requirements for
iron and other anemia-preventing nutrients is increased
during periods of stress, such as rapid growth periods
during infancy and adolescence, and in the childbearing
years in women. It is difficult to adjust the diet to meet
these circumstances. Not only is the need for iron increased, but the need for folic acid, vitamin B-6, vitamin B-12 and protein as well.

Magnitude of Benefits From Nutritional Research*

Health Problem	Magnitude	Potential savings from improved diet
Heart and Vascular Disorders	Over 1,000,000 deaths in 1967.	25% reduction
Respiratory and Infectious Diseases	141 million workdays lost in 1965-66; 166 million school days lost.	15-20% fewer lost days.
Mental Health	5.2 million people are severely or totally disabled; 25 million have manifest disability.	10% fewer disabilities.
Early Aging	About 49.1% of population have one or more chronic impairments: 102 million people.	10 million people without impairments.
Problems of Reproduction	15 million with congenital birth defects.	3 million fewer children with birth defects.
Arthritis	16 million afflicted.	8 million people without afflictions.
Dental Health	50% of all people over 55 have no teeth; $6.5 billion public and private expenditures on dentists' services in 1967.	50% reduction in incidence, severity and expenditures.
Diabetes and Carbohydrate Disorders	3.9 million overt diabetic deaths in 1967; 79% of people over 55 with impaired glucose tolerance.	50% of cases avoided or improved.

*Human Nutrition Report 2. Science and Education Staff of USDA. August, 1971.

Health Problem	Magnitude	Potential savings from improved diet
Osteoporosis	4 million severe cases; 25% of women over 40.	75% reduction
Obesity	30 to 40% of adults; 60 to 70% over 40 years.	75% reduction
Alcoholism	10 million alcoholics; 50% are addicted; annual loss over $2 billion from absenteeism, lowered production and accidents.	33% reduction
Problems of Eyesight	48.1% or 86 million people over 3 years wore corrective lenses in 1966; 81,000 became blind every year; 103 million on welfare.	20% fewer people blind or with corrective lenses.
Allergies	22 million people (9%) are allergic; 16 million with hayfever or asthma; 7-15 million people allergic to milk.	20% of people relieved; 90% of those allergic to milk.
Digestive Disorders	About 20 million incidents of acute condition annually; 4,000 new cases each day; 14 million with duodenal ulcers.	25% fewer acute conditions; over $1 billion in costs.
Kidney and Urinary Diseases	55,000 deaths from renal failure; 200,000 with kidney stones.	20% reduction in incidence and deaths.
Musclar Disorders	200,000 cases.	10% reduction in cases.
Cancer	600,000 persons developed cancer in 1968; 320,000 persons died of cancer in 1968.	20% reduction in incidence and deaths.

Improved Growth and Development	324.5 million workdays lost; 51.8 million people needing medical attention and/or restricted activity.	25% fewer work days lost.
Improved Learning Ability	Over 6.5 million mentally retarded with I.Q. below 70; 12% of school-age children need special education.	I.Q. raised by 10 points for persons with I.Q. 70-80.

About ten million persons in this country are alcoholics according to conservative estimates. This is a disease of the metabolism in which neurological manifestations become dominant. It is characterized by deficient diets, usually brought on by lack of appetite or actual inability to partake adequately of wholesome foods because of a nervous reaction which interferes with the mechanics of swallowing them. As a result, alcoholics tend to exist largely on the empty calories of alcoholic drinks.

Wholesome foods which can provide vitamin B-6, pantothenic acid, magnesium and vitamin B-1—all necessary for normal nerve function—may be grossly lacking. Protein deficiency is almost universal among this group. A recent report relates that soft drink addicts may follow a pattern similar to the alcoholic in substituting empty calories for wholesome foods. If this group is added to the other groups which are excessively devoted to diets in which empty calories predominate, a considerable proportion of our total population is represented. Such habits may be difficult to change without the assistance provided by a well-planned nutritional supplementation program. The USDA report comments as follows:

"There is now some evidence with rats [test animals] that craving for alcohol [and we assume soft drinks] can result from a chemical imbalance created by inadequate diet. Switching to a well-balanced diet was accompanied by a [voluntary] reduction in alcohol consumption."

The complete title of the USDA report is *An Evaluation of Research in the United States on Human Nutrition Report 2: Prepared by a joint group of the U.S. Department of Agriculture and the state universities and land grant colleges.* This report makes some very unusual evaluations in regard to present conditions of health and what improved nutrition can be expected to accomplish for them. These evaluations are qualified by the following statement:

"Estimates of potential savings are judgments based on review of scientific literature and discussions with clinicians. No claim is made that all of the benefits are included or that the claim made for nutrition's contribution to the problems are as great or small as eventually may be realized. At best they are subjective evaluations, because basic data do not exist."

Yes, it is true: Some people do need vitamins more than others, and if indications of the USDA report quoted are taken into account, "some people" includes just about everybody.

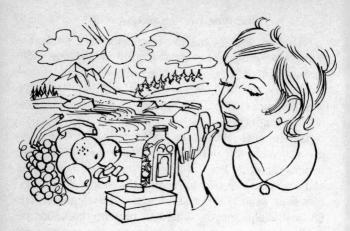

Chapter V

BASIC SUPPLEMENTS

WHAT IS a food supplement? I once heard of a case where a criminal entered a plea of not guilty to passing counterfeit money on the basis that there was no such thing, saying "If it's counterfeit, it's not money, and if it's money, it's not counterfeit."

An analogy can be made with food supplements. Foods, according to *Taber's Medical Dictionary*, are "nutritive substances necessary to nourish, protect and maintain the body." A supplement is "something added to make up for a deficiency or to reinforce." Natural foods with all their perfection, do not, of course, need to be supplemented in this sense, and if they are not complete and balanced in themselves we adopt the term Protective Dietary Nutriments instead of the commonly used term food supplements, which for many people has lost its meaning.

There are some half-hundred nutritive substances that can come under the PDN (Protective Dietary Nutriment) classification. This includes not only the essential vitamins and minerals ("essential" meaning necessary for life or growth), but also many functional foods, which although not essential do perform many needed and useful nutritional tasks.

These last include such food factors as lecithin, bioflavonoids, choline, rutin, acetic acid (vinegar), enzymes, kelp, yeast, pectin and many others. Another group of PDN substances are those included under the herbal food classification, including such herbs as ginseng, fenugreek, thyme, golden seal and many others too numerous to mention here.

A third group of PDN substances are those used for intestinal hygienic purposes. These include natural adsorbents, such as colloidal mineral complexes, and carminatives such as fennel and natural orthophosphoric acid, as well as the slowly absorbed sugar lactose, which acts as a food for favorable bacteria in the colon. By raising our sights from the mere "good supplement class" and including the PDN potentials in the picture, we obtain a much clearer view of what the modern nutritional perspective is all about.

There are various vehicles used to make food supplements or PDN's more convenient and easier and more efficient to use. They may be in the form of tablets, capsules, gelatin perles, liquid or powder. Potent drugs are administered in the same forms although the ingredients are entirely different. Still, many persons have a mental block when it comes to swallowing what they call "pills," even though one kind is health-building and the other may be a risk to health. This is important, particularly when a large number of tablets or capsules must be taken in order to provide nutritionally effective amounts of some PDN nutrients. This is especially true insofar as minerals are concerned, which are required in much larger amounts than vitamins.

For example, you can easily get all of the essential vitamins required for normal nutrition in one tablet, but it might take 10 or 12 tablets to provide the equivalent nutritional needs for minerals. There is only so much space in a tablet and different nutrients take up varying amounts of space. To illustrate, one milligram of vitamin B-1 as compared to about 750 milligrams of calcium are the proportionate space (weight) required in a tablet for these two essential nutrients.

We have also become confused by the maze of semantics (interpretation of words) used to describe nutritional products. We commonly hear such terms as "natural," and "organic" used. What do they actually mean? It depends upon who uses the term. To the scientist or technician, the word "organic" means a compound containing the carbon molecule; to a health-minded nutritional advocate, organic means something which is inborn or coming from life (both meanings are listed in Webster's). As to the word "natural," its meaning is quite clear: "according to nature." Superimpose on these terms the word "synthetic" and the confusion increases even further. Synthetic also has two meanings according to who is using the term.

To the scientist synthesizing simply means "putting together of parts or elements to form a whole" (the opposite of analyzing or taking apart); but to the nutrition-minded person "synthetic" means "artificial, not real or genuine" (both definitions from Webster). This confusion is further compounded by the fact that labeling laws require that nutrients listed must, in many cases, show their chemical names, regardless of their source. Vitamin B-1 must be designated as thiamin, B-2 as riboflavin, and so forth.

In addition, labeling laws require all sorts of technical jargon which acts to confuse the reader further, such as "minimum adult daily requirements," "MDR not established," "Need in human nutrition has not been established," until, in fact, it takes practically a skilled Food and Drug Administration lawyer to understand an ordinary food supplement label.

Is there any way you can put these parts together and come up with reasoning which will fit your good judgment and common sense? I think there is. I wish to introduce a new term for describing PDN formulations. Let us describe them as *segregated nutriments*. This term can satisfy all of those who use the words "natural," "synthetic," or "organic." It will allow the nutritionist to select the most advantageous formulation of his products—to use formulas which can and do correct the nutritional difficulties so prevalent in our times. He will feel free to recommend inorganic minerals (which are essential to life); he will feel free to recommend nutritive factors which have been duplicated from nature, when necessary, in the laboratory; he will be able to utilize modern scientific knowledge because all of its tools will be available, without having to wear blinders simply because certain words are being misused or misinterpreted.

We will not have lost one whit by this step forward! "Natural" still means "according to nature"; "synthetic" still means "put together to form a whole"; "organic" still means "of, relating to, or derived from living organisms" (all living things contain the carbon molecule). What we will have gained is a clearer understanding of the terms we use and by offering a more compatible expression—"segregated nutriments"—have a much firmer and still scientific foundation upon which to stand.

In the final analysis, the person who uses food and food products properly to improve his health is the final judge of their effectiveness. Their effect in a practical situation is the only "acid test" that can be applied. Learn to trust your own ability to observe and feel results; fortify your knowledge with literature and articles and be confident that in the long run you will be enjoying a more healthful, more active and longer life.

HOW IONS KEEP THE HUMAN BATTERY CHARGED

Blink your eye, move your finger, think about what you are reading—none of these would be possible without an electrical reaction within your body. It is the same kind of electricity that starts your car, toasts your bread and lights your home. It differs only in amount. The actual quantity of electricity in your body is so small that extremely delicate instruments are used to measure it; yet this tiny bit of electricity exerts a tremendous force in the regulation of bodily functions.

The question arises: How can such a minute quantity of electricity be made to perform such a prodigious amount of work? An off-the-cuff answer might be: Through the nervous system. But this does not explain where the nervous system gets the electricity it needs to operate with in the first place. As a matter of fact, electricity in the body goes far beyond the nervous system itself and actually penetrates into the smallest units of life, the cell. Each of the cells—about 100 trillion of them—has within it its own electrical charge. And, when we realize that about a billion new cells are born to us every hour, the importance of keeping these cells charged becomes a major consideration in matters pertaining to our health.

The key to understanding this phenomenon is in the field of physical chemistry which is called "ionization." The word need not confuse you. It is not difficult to understand. Ionization is simply the process by which molecules accumulate positive or negative electrical charges. A simple illustration of ionization is static electricity. This can be caused by friction, such as walking on a fibrous carpet, then is discharged by touching the metal knob of a door. But within the body itself another kind of ionization occurs. This is the kind which occurs when minerals are put into a watery medium. It is dependent upon the minerals losing certain molecules to the water so that they are free from their original compound.

In other words, when salt is put into water, a number of free sodium and free chloride molecules go into solution. These free molecules take on either positive or negative charges according to their chemical nature. This can be demonstrated by the process of hydrolysis of water which occurs at a much faster rate if salt is present in the solution. The experiment is made by placing a positive and negative electrode in a tank of distilled water. Hydrogen comes off one electrode, oxygen off the other.

In distilled water the reaction is slow, but when salt is added the rate rapidly accelerates. The sodium and chloride ions act as "electrical hands" which speed up the reaction.

In a similar manner, ions in the body keep the "human battery" charged. But in this case, not only do sodium and chloride become ionized (as in our tank experiment), but also a number of other minerals and substances. The most important of these are potassium, calcium, phosphorus and magnesium, but amino acids and many radicals (chemical combinations) can also assume the ionized state.

An important thing to remember about ions is that they can assume only one kind of charge: it must be either positive or negative. Both kinds must be present for physiological balance. Technically, this is referred to as "ionic equilibrium." The terminology used by physicians to describe the method used to reestablish ionic equilibrium is "electrolyte therapy." Such treatment marks one of the greatest advancements modern medicine has made in physiological medicine. Many lives have been saved by dripping these human battery recharging elements into the blood stream from a bottle hung over a hospital bed.

The trouble is that this method of treatment is largely restricted to situations which require lifesaving measures. That is a shame. The same life-giving elements which doctors call "electrolytes" are contained in foods we should eat every day. In plain language, they are *minerals*. It is true that an ounce of prevention is worth a pound of cure, and nowhere does that adage apply so appropriately as here.

Many people neglect supplementing their diet with minerals simply because they do not know that they are necessary to keep the human battery charged. There is not an essential mineral that does not contribute to this effect. Each works in a different way (producing either positive or negative charges, for example), but like spokes in a wheel they all support the main function. When all spokes are present, and in the proper quantities, we have the desirable state of being in ionic equilibrium; when one or more is lacking, discord and imbalance results and our health is affected.

A common way of expressing such an imbalance is

to describe it as either acidosis or alkalosis (meaning a state of reduced or increased acidity or alkalinity of the blood and tissues, due to excessive or deficient quantities of acid or alkaline minerals. But the correction of either condition per se is not a simple matter as often the treatment itself can result in furthering the imbalance and laymen and doctors alike are often confused by the subject. Rather than approaching the problem on an acid-alkaline basis, it is much better to provide the complete pattern of mineral elements in the diet and allow nature to take over the balancing job.

Nature usually does this quite well. In fact we have a term to describe the process. It is called "homeostasis," which simply means that, given the materials it needs to work with, nature will act to maintain the body within the narrow limits of its normal metabolism.

The next question to be asked is: Is the average American getting enough minerals in his diet? This is easy to answer, but difficult to prove by referring to present-day scientific facts on the subject. Textbooks frequently treat the subject of mineral deficiency according to concepts which have been outdated by modern findings. We are told by the books, for example, that a well-balanced diet provides sufficient potassium and magnesium while, in reality, doctors are prescribing these minerals for patients in a host of conditions ranging from heart disease to nervous disorders.

The subject of magnesium deficiency is of current scientific interest and many such investigations have given cause to suspect that it is much more severe and widespread than formerly suspected. In Asiatic countries, for example, where hardening of the arteries and associated heart disease is relatively rare, blood analysis shows ample magnesium, while in this country where such disease is common, similar analyses show a much lower level of this essential mineral. The truth is that there are many known reasons why a common mineral deficiency may be suspected.

What are the factors which contribute to a deficient mineral intake in the diet? Paradoxically, a high protein diet—as good as it is in itself—increases the need for potassium which is important in protein metabolism. Disturbances in carbohydrate metabolism (from diabetes to hypoglycemia) are also associated with the need for potassium. The consumption of milk (our principle source of calcium) is intolerable for many lactose-intolerant people.

Most people could not name even one food rich in magnesium, so how could you expect them to select a diet rich in this nutrient? Boiling foods in water leaches them of minerals (which are water-soluble) and the water is then thrown away. The USDA tells us that one-third of the minerals in canned foods is in the water, for example. People who eat in restaurants are at a particular disadvantage. Often even the most high-priced meals in exclusive restaurants feature only the high protein foods (steak, lobster, shrimp) on their menus, while the vegetable portions served at the same meal may be a sham. Of course, it is obvious that the refined foods, such as white bread and white sugar, are either completely devoid of minerals or so stripped of their original mineral content that they can only be called "anemic" in this regard.

One reason why mineral deficiency has become the American affliction is that minerals can not be made into food supplements that are as convenient to take as vitamins. Vitamins are microfactors in food and, being small, many vitamins can be included in a simple tablet which can be taken on a one- or two-per-day basis. Vitamin-and-mineral formulas have minerals in them, which is helpful, but to get the minerals in the quantities you really need, special formulations are involved. In this respect, one or two mineral supplements a day (of calcium, potassium and magnesium in particular) may be little better than not taking this kind of supplement at all. The estimated requirement for potassium, for example, is between 1,500 and 2,000 milligrams per day, for calcium about 750 milligrams a day, and an estimated daily requirement for magnesium is between 300 and 400 milligrams a day. So figure it out for yourself: more tablets are needed for minerals than for vitamins. It is just that simple.

So how can one go about supplementing the diet with minerals themselves? Drink one or two glasses of vegetable juice every day (it is rich in potassium as well as other nutrients) or take a food supplement in which adequate minerals are provided. To help your body assimilate minerals better, stop eating refined foods, such as white flour and white sugar and use salt moderately (sodium in salt is one mineral we can get too much of but, unless it is restricted by a doctor, we need some sodium too). Above all, eat a diet high in garden vegetables (uncooked preferably) to keep your human battery charged—that's the best way of all.

BASIC SUPPLEMENTS

I have been asked so frequently for a basic program of supplementation for the average individual (not for one who is ill or has a problem) that I think the time has come for such a program to be outlined. It must be kept in mind that each of us is an individual with different needs as far as supplementation is concerned. However, the program that follows is one that I use as a maintenance program for my family and myself, and which I regularly recommend to persons who are interested in getting a little extra insurance for their daily diet.

BASIC NUMBER ONE

Everyone should take a good natural organic multiple vitamin and mineral supplement. Because of advertising, and suggestions by many physicians, few persons will dispute the good sense in taking a multiple vitamin-mineral supplement, but there the agreement ends. The hue and cry of various commercial and governmental agencies would have you believe that a synthetic vitamin and a natural vitamin are identical in action in the human body. Let us consider, first of all, what a vitamin is. It is a complex mechanism of biological "wheels within wheels." It may consist of enzymes, coenzymes, enzyme activators and antioxidant protective factors. Since enzymes are protein in nature, they must contain amino acids and trace minerals. Enzyme activators may include manganese, cobalt, vanadium and molybdenum—all of which are probably effective only when present in the proper soluble state.

Enzyme activity is destroyed by the heat of pasteurization temperatures. A vitamin that has been subjected to such crude treatment is as much a vitamin as an auto is after it has smashed into a brick wall at 100 mph. I should warn you that the preceding statement is strictly my own opinion and is in conflict with governmental and medical consensus. The vitamin may remain the same chemically, but functionally it will not react the same or produce the same results.

It therefore behooves the thinking individual to consider the source of the vitamin preparations he is taking. Many ultra-high-potency vitamins are of a synthetic origin and should be recognized as such. Vitamins

from natural sources are often segregated by crysta
tion to achieve a higher potency, a necessary and acc
able procedure. While the average body does not need
high potency, it does require a complex of natural ingredients to furnish all the synergistic factors which make a
vitamin effective. This has been brought out clearly,
time after time. Failure often results when we think we
recognize a deficiency and attempt to treat it by adding
only one particular substance of the diet. Pernicious
anemia is an example—iron alone is not enough; vitamin B-12 is also needed. Research is now indicating
that in treating any anemia an adequate amount of vitamin C must be present or all the iron and liver and
B-complex in the world will fail to produce a response.

Five per cent of the whole body consists of mineral
matter. These minerals are essential to life and the absence of them in the diet would result in death. Certain
habits, either in the food pattern or in dissipation, can
so deplete certain minerals as to bring about a deficiency
and the symptoms thereof. In other instances, a lack of
synergistic material may hinder the proper utilization of
a certain mineral, bringing about a deficiency.

Vitamins have often been compared with the delicate adjustments necessary by a skilled mechanic to
tune up your car. Minerals, in the same light, are like
the parts that fit together to make the machinery of the
body run. Without minerals—no matter how skilled the
"mechanic"—he is working with defective parts and no
amount of "adjustments" can give a proper tune-up
and flawless performance.

It is my practice to recommend a medium potency
multiple vitamin-mineral formula of natural organic
origin at the rate of about four-per-day, preferably in a
split dose. This vitamin-mineral complex should also

include vitamins A, D and B-complex plus the minerals.

BASIC NUMBER TWO

The "C" of Life

Much has been said and written of the various food factors by nutritional scientists and researchers. They do not always agree as to the need of certain substances in human nutrition but there is very little, if any, dissension when it comes to vitamin C. This is the most fragile and perishable of all natural vitamins—dissolving easily in water and greatly diminished by exposure to air or sunlight. Many years ago, a strange fact came to light: Although vitamin C is found in every living cell and in every plant and animal organism, man seems to have been singled out by nature as one of the few living creatures unable to build this essential life-giving element within himself. He is dependent upon a continual sustaining intake of vitamin C in his diet.

This important vitamin has a long history; the anti-scurvy factor in fresh oranges and lemons was reported as early as 1593 by Sir Richard Hawkins of the British Royal Navy. But it took the simple remedy of pine needle tea used by the American Indian and demonstrated to Jacques Cartier, the discoverer of Canada, to bring about a more general awareness of this factor found only in fresh fruits or vegetables. Even then, the advocates of carrying lemon juice on board ship met with scoffers, and with those who claimed that the drinking of lemon juice did not prevent scurvy because they had lemon juice aboard their ship and scurvy incidence was just as high as any other time. Investigation of this report turned up the interesting fact that the lemon juice had been boiled for long periods of time in order that it might "retain its effectiveness." Fortunately, this factor was correctly interpreted and the juice was no longer "processed." Later, the British Royal Navy made it mandatory for each man to have his daily portion of lemon juice while at sea. Many historians credit this with giving Britain undisputed command of the seas for so many years, while men in other navies sickened and died. Scurvy was a rampant disease in that era and not always confined to sailors. Symptoms were quite easy to determine as the disease followed a definite course: bleeding of the gums and inflammation, then loosening of the teeth followed by internal hemorrhages, anemia and dropsy. The introduction of the potato to Europe is credited with aiding in the elimination of the disease, particularly in impoverished areas where the diet was limited. This is amply borne out by the outbreak of scurvy in Ireland in 1846, the year of the potato crop failure.

The properties of vitamin C are so diversified that it is difficult to list all of them, but the dominant factors are as follows.

The most important (and many times overlooked) characteristic is the cohesive or cementing action of vitamin C. Here it acts to hold the cells of the body together; the walls of the arteries, veins and capillaries, the ligaments, cartilages and matrices of the bones are all dependent on this vitamin for their firmness. If insufficient vitamin C is present, the walls become pulpy and watery and minerals spill out and are excreted. The resultant mineral loss can be extremely dangerous in acute disease.

There is a fantastic amount of clinical evidence available as to the value of vitamin C in almost every type of infective disorder as well as many disorders not normally considered in this category, e.g., as a protective factor against sunburn, poison ivy, chicken pox, measles, mumps, herpes zoster (shingles) and arthritic-rheumatoid states.

It is extremely important to keep the body saturated with vitamin C during any stress or strain. Since vitamin C is not stored in the body, a continued dosage is of utmost importance when an acute situation is at hand. In this way, the body always has some of this important substance available.

Vitamin C can truthfully be designated as the antitoxin and antiviral vitamin. By combining with the toxins and the virus invaders, the vitamin renders them powerless and quickens the recovery period. Many learned authorities have reported similar effects with high-dosage vitamin C as are obtained with sulfa or the antibiotics.

Vitamin C is considered necessary for pregnant or nursing mothers and essential for infant feeding.

Vitamin C is closely related to proper functioning of the adrenal gland and the production of cortisone so necessary for proper function of the body; indirectly, it increases gamma globulin by increasing antibody formation. Because of its relationship to the adrenal gland, it has been used successfully in the treatment of severe burns; the adrenals are the first glands to respond to burns and an inadequate response can seriously delay recovery. Many surgeons are now using vitamin C both pre- and postoperatively to accelerate tissue repair and recuperation.

Although the American Medical Association maintains that there is no nutritional problem in the United States except in those rare instances in which a doctor diagnoses malnutrition, nation-wide surveys and studies would indicate that on a high school level, more than 46 percent of the students are frequently deficient in vitamin C. When individual groups such as college coeds were catalogued, the fantastic figure of 82 percent deficiency was reported, utilizing the minimum adult daily requirement as the standard. In addition to this, let us consider the individual who smokes. Clinical evidence would seem to prove that every cigarette depletes the body of 25 mg of vitamin C. If this is so, the minimum daily adult requirement of 30 mg jumps to 530 mg per day for the one pack a day smoker. Stresses and strain can increase the body's need for vitamin C just as much or more than smoking, hence the 30 mg figure is truly a minimum requirement.

In nature, vitamin C is usually found in combination with bioflavonoid complex and rutin, two other nutritional factors which are complementary and synergistic with vitamin C. It is an unfortunate but true fact that researchers will often discover great pearls of wisdom only to be mocked and degraded by others because they could not duplicate the results. Too often such failures result because the substance used in the experiments was not exactly the same. This has occurred in the use of vitamin C complexes as found in nature (containing the bioflavonoids and rutin) when compared to the chemically produced ascorbic acid also known as vitamin C but lacking the other factors.

If I described all the seemingly miraculous occurrences following the use of vitamin C with its appropriate synergists, I might be accused of being over-enthusiastic and unrealistic; however, medical literature is full of documented reports and your awareness of such a simple remedy covering such a broad spectrum can mean much to your health picture. Common foodstuffs which contain quality vitamin C are: green peppers, mung bean sprouts, broccoli, kohlrabi, raw cabbage, parsley, apples, tomatoes, strawberries, oranges, lemons, fresh guava, watercress and cauliflower. Recommended dosages vary from 500 to 5000 or more milligrams per day, although a happy medium of about 2500 mg seems to be adequate for average use. Extra dosage does not bring about toxic side effects so be safe by using a little extra.

BASIC NUMBER THREE

Vitamin E is the most widely sold and used of all vitamins at this time, due in great part to excellent books and articles concerning research on this substance. However, we again must consider where the true facts lie since we can buy vitamin E in so many forms, in so many potencies and in a wide price range.

The hue and cry of the past few years has settled down in respect to vitamin E and its use in the armamentaria of medicine. Not too many years ago vitamin E was finally accepted as a necessary factor in human nutrition but a minimum daily requirement was not established. In order to understand how orthodox medicine can pass by or brush aside a substance as fascinating and exciting therapeutically as vitamin E, you must remember that the average practitioner of medicine is so overwhelmed with taking care of the acute symptoms of disease that he has little time for personal observation or research. His tools, primarily drugs, are those which he learned about in school or those which the journal of his association recommends as being efficacious. He should not be condemned for being caught in a whirlwind not of his own making but that of a mode of life which has given rise to an octopus-like structure controlling all within its sphere.

When vitamin E was first accepted as an essential

part of the human diet, the advocates of its use thought they had won a great battle, but instead they found the victory shallow indeed. Before acceptance as a necessity, many books were written about vitamin E, clinical data was pursued with vigor and people extolled its virtue at every opportunity. Now we find that peace and calm have descended over these individuals and they have found other battles to engage in. New research is limited and crusading publications are almost nonexistent. I feel obligated at this time to submit my views and observations on a remarkable food factor which, although considered essential for life, is sadly lacking in the average diet.

It is an interesting coincidence that about the same time that the millers of flour decided that removing the bran and germ of the wheat would give them a product which had a much longer shelf life, scientists were working with an unknown substance which prevented fetal resorption in animals which had been fed a rancid lard diet; the substance was labeled vitamin E. It has taken many years for the realization to come about that the removal of the germ of the wheat also removed the vitamin E content and that the resulting white flour was an inferior product nutritionally because of this loss.

It did not take long for the hucksters to promote the idea that the whiter the flour or sugar the more pure and clean it was. Children were brought up with the idea firmly entrenched in their minds that the dark breads and raw sugars were dirty and undesirable. I might add that it takes a great deal of rationalization to overcome these prejudices. In our present day, few families use whole grain breads or whole wheat products in their homes. Since this is one of the staple sources of vitamin E, it has become increasingly apparent that the average daily intake of vitamin E in our diet is low. Various studies have been made throughout the years on vitamin E deficiencies, but they were mostly concerned with the original concept of an adequate supply preventing abortions and fetal resorptions.

The linking of the process of reproduction and vitamin E deficiency overshadowed some of the more valuable and significant properties of this substance as well as probably causing the Food and Drug Administration to look with a jaundiced eye upon any claims for rejuvenation. Such claims are considered unethical in any profession and the rather exorbitant claims made by the unscrupulous acted as a deterrent to proper evaluation of vitamin E for many years.

Now that this vitamin is a recognized essential in the human diet pattern, many different products are available for the consumer. This could be confusing to some because of the variety offered, so let's take a look at what vitamin E consists of and what to look for in a potential product. First of all, it should be clearly understood that much of the recognized research which produced results in test animals used a wheat germ oil introduced by mouth into the body. Several papers were written about the seeming lack of results when the substance was introduced by other means. Just as in the history of vitamin C, the scientist is always curious as to just what factor in the wheat germ oil brings about these reactions. Soon the term "tocopherol" was coined and then broken down into alpha, beta, gamma and delta fractions. (Interestingly enough, "tocopherol" literally translated from the Greek language means "to bring forth childbirth" and yet this is the least important of its functions.) When the finding was published that the alpha tocopherol factor seemed to be the most active, emphasis was immediately shifted to this substance.

Now the controversy rages as to whether it is even necessary to include the other tocopherols in a vitamin E preparation. Some excellent work done by a group of doctors would seem to indicate that alpha tocopherol is a boon to heart patients, but a closer study indicates its limitations and contraindications. According to this report, certain types of heart conditions do not respond to alpha tocopherol application and its use may even aggravate the condition. I have used the mixed tocopherols for many years in all kinds of heart cases and have never seen a side effect or contraindication. This has been amply researched by many other scientists and we must come back to the old adage—"It is not possible to improve on nature." There is always the necessity for the complex of substances found in nature to be present in order to accomplish the complete work.

The same applies to attempts to make the vitamin E preparation more palatable by processing out the oils, because some people may have unpleasant gastrointestinal sensations when taking an oil-soluble product. If only we would heed the warnings of nature, we would realize this is only a sign that the liver is not functioning properly and attention should be temporarily given to this organ. I have found that using lecithin in the same capsule or in addition to the vitamin E will usually take care of the problem as lecithin is an excellent emulsifier of oils.

High potency advocates are of the opinion that the individual intake should be from 400 to 1000 IUs per day. I have found this to be true providing that the complete complex of tocopherols is given. Certain situations may call for larger quantities initially, but these can usually be reduced. As a general rule, I recommend 400 to 1000 IUs of d-alpha tocopherol in a base of wheat germ oil and lecithin per day (remember, dl-alpha tocopherol is a synthetic preparation and has not demonstrated the same effect that d-alpha has) in conjunction with a diet including some of the whole grains. Wheat germ oil provides the mixed tocopherols naturally.

Since we have not even spoken of the other properties of vitamin E, let us discuss the one which is most important. Vitamin E acts as an anti-oxidant, which is to say that it inhibits or slows down oxidation. Oxidation is the natural enemy of many substances, particularly foodstuffs, because after oxidation deterioration begins. It has been demonstrated that a deficiency of vitamin E can cause enzyme systems to go awry. It is not completely clear whether the E enters into the enzyme reaction or whether it acts as a protector by being an anti-oxidant. I prefer the latter approach because of the fact that as vitamin E is introduced throughout the body, you find a decrease in the oxidative mechanism. As an effective anti-oxidant vitamin E is probably one of the most broadly applicable of the vitamins in any degenerative disease. It has been used with salutary effects in diabetes, muscular dystrophy, stress and old age, indolent and peptic ulcers, varicose veins, kidney and liver diseases and the entire spectrum of cardiovascular disturbances.

The seemingly miraculous healing benefits observed daily by adherents of vitamin E have created certain problems. There is nothing the scientific community dislikes more than the approval of and devotion to what it considers unscientific experiments. Vitamin E enthusiasts, particularly those who have been brought back from the life of an invalid to once again become active, functioning human beings, do tend to become something akin to zealots.

I personally can attest to many instances when seriously ill heart patients made remarkable recoveries after undergoing vitamin E therapy, but the attending physicians refused to credit such use as even a contributing factor to the healing; diabetic ulcers that had resisted all efforts by allopathic medicine were healed by the external application of a vitamin E ointment and integral use of 800 IUs daily; and the same vitamin E ointment time after time brought relief from third-degree burns within twenty-four hours after being applied.

In summary, vitamin E offers a broad spectrum of application with no known side effects if the mixed oil-soluble tocopherols are used. In order to facilitate assimilation, an emulsifying factor such as lecithin can be used. Dosage will vary but for preventive and maintenance purposes, 400 to 1000 IUs per day of a high quality product would seem adequate (this does not apply in therapeutic cases, of course). I hope that this wonder substance will one day find its proper place in the prevention and treatment of chronic degenerative diseases.

BASIC NUMBER FOUR

Although calcium is a rather common element in our daily diet, calcium deficiency remains one of the prevalent nutritional deficiencies. There are myriad calcium products on the market, many of which are very good. It is my observation that the soluble calcium, free of phosphorus, is the most needed. This type of calcium cooperates well with vitamin C to control infections and combat such symptoms as canker sores, fever and fever blisters and cold sores. Taken on an empty stomach, it is effective in controlling muscle cramps and enhancing muscle relaxation during menstruation and in instances of insomnia.

The mineral magnesium must also be combined with such calcium for proper utilization. I also feel that small amounts of vitamin C and either betaine hydrochloride or glutamic acid hydrochloride are necessary to make sure that the calcium is assimilated. It must be emphasized that we are speaking of a calcium which will be primarily used by muscle and nerve tissue; the calcium taken in during the normal course of eating is primarily used as bone calcium.

I take a calcium-magnesium supplement which yields approximately 2000 mg calcium and about 800-plus mg magnesium. A little hydrochloric acid from some source aids many to assimilate and utilize this calcium. I feel this balances and supplements my calcium intake adequately.

The preceding basic program will not meet with the approval of all readers. Some will say, "How about kelp" or any other number of substances. Let me assure you that any good multiple vitamin-mineral preparation will include kelp, and probably a dozen other substances that are commonly used alone. I only hope that my suggestions will serve as guidelines for those who are sincerely considering a concise food supplement program.

SUMMARY

Basic Number One:
Always take a good multiple food supplement with a natural base and source.

Basic Number Two:
Use extra vitamin C up to 3000 mg daily.

Basic Number Three:
   Vitamin E from 400 to 1000 IU or more daily, preferably with lecithin.

Basic Number Four:
   Add from 1500-2000 mg calcium with magnesium to your daily fare.

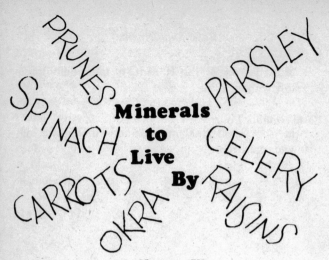

PRUNES PARSLEY SPINACH CELERY Minerals to Live By CARROTS OKRA RAISINS

Chapter VI

MINERALS TO LIVE BY

So MANY times I have heard the question, "Doctor, what foods should I eat for certain mineral deficiencies? I read an article the other day and I have all the signs of a calcium [or any other mineral] lack in my body." People like to experiment a little on their own so I am going to give a thumbnail sketch of the various minerals, their primary functions in the body and the foods which contain an appreciable amount of each. It will be impossible for me to be complete as this is a field all its own.

Let us start with the most popular—calcium. A deficiency of this mineral can cause poor bone formation, decayed teeth, irritability, excessive perspiration, nervousness, worry, susceptibility to colds, and a constant feeling of exhaustion.

Experts will tell you that there are so many sources

of calcium in our daily foods that it would be almost impossible to have a deficiency. The fallacy in this thinking is that for the proper utilization of calcium several other factors must also be present—fatty acids, the enzyme phosphatase, and sufficient digestive juices to break it down. In addition, it is now thought that vitamin C plays a role in calcium utilization, as does magnesium. In some instances, because of a lack of these synergistic materials, there is a loss of calcium in the form of calcium oxalates, which some authorities believe has a direct effect upon such conditions as arthritis, gallstones, hardening of the arteries and joint stiffness. This is possible because the body, if it is not able to excrete or utilize the calcium, will deposit it somewhere. Good sources of calcium are raw milk, egg yolk, turnip greens, asparagus, beans, cauliflower and almonds.

Iron deficiency corresponds to anemia, low vitality, decreased red blood cells, pale complexion, dry mouth and red tongue. Synergistic factors are copper, hydrochloric acid, cobalt or vitamin B-12. In the absence of any of these factors, sufficient iron may be ingested but cannot be utilized. Foods high in iron are spinach, raisins, almonds, bran, dates, figs, apricots, molasses and parsley.

The mineral phosphorus unites with many other minerals (including calcium, sodium, iron and magnesium) in order to create healthy bones, nerve fibers, brain and red blood cells. A deficiency is shown by retarded growth, mental or physical, accompanied by over-excitability or apparent stupidity. There is often a loss of weight, rickets and defective cell activity. One of the more important subclinical signs of this deficiency is a lack of ability to concentrate sufficiently to carry out any task to a successful conclusion.

Phosphorus is found in egg yolk, raw milk, lecithin, barley, oatmeal, peanuts, peas, whole wheat and rye, lentils, walnuts, beans and bran.

Sodium (not to be construed to mean sodium chloride or common table salt) is a very important mineral in the body, being necessary to preserve a balance between calcium and potassium to maintain normal heart action and the equilibrium of the body. It aids in regulating the osmotic pressure in the cells necessary to stop the excessive loss of water from the tissues. Deficiency of sodium leads to acidosis, deafness, catarrh, stiffness of the joints and constipation.

Sodium is found in okra, celery, spinach, carrots, apples, prunes, raw turnips, string beans, asparagus, figs, peaches, oats, beets, cucumbers and lamb. One should try to obtain sodium from these sources rather than sodium chloride because the excessive use of the latter product can be just as injurious to the system as a lack of sodium.

A few of the symptoms of excessive sodium chloride intake are: exhaustion type headache, hangnails, dry hair and skin, high blood pressure, anemia and irritability. There seems to be a correlation between excessive salt eating and a vitriolic temper.

Potassium is an alkaline mineral which works closely with sodium to maintain the ionic balance in the system. It is known to be necessary for normal growth but until recently, doctors were not necessarily aware of the various disorders associated with potassium deficiency. Disorders of the nervous system, loss of weight, poor digestion, irregular heart action and poor muscular control are all now considered to be associated with low potassium levels in the human. Excellent sources of this mineral are: bran, beans, olives, molasses, spinach, raisins, parsnips, potatoes, apricots, asparagus, beets, cabbage and carrots.

The trace minerals are coming more and more to the front in nutrition now. Mineral elements such as manganese, copper, zinc, cobalt, silicon and many others are now considered to be as important as the more familiar ones. It is a rather interesting fact that the many trace elements found in the sea—which is actually composed of all the elements known to man—are duplicated in the human system on an almost identical percentage basis. Some authorities have indicated that because of this the ingestion of sea water could be of benefit to the human system. It could prove to be an economical and balanced way of aiding the body to balance its mineral chemistry.

MINERALS—UNSUNG HEROES OF LIFE

Of all the essential nutrients, minerals have received the least attention of scientific investigators. More often than not, you can read a scientific textbook on nutrition with chapter after chapter on the intricacies of vitamin uses only to find the discussion of minerals jammed into a few meager pages at the back of the book. Why this neglect of these important nutritive elements?

For one thing, minerals have been recognized as essential to human nutrition since long before vitamins were discovered. The vitamin era started to bloom about 70 years ago at the turn of the century. They captured the imagination of scientist and lay person alike and have held the spotlight ever since. Minerals have been treated as a "go along" thing, their presence rather casually taken for granted.

A dramatic development in scientific circles changed

that outlook among doctors and physicians, but the discovery has failed to filter down to the public. This
method of therapy began with the Ringer experiments
discussed earlier in this work. To refresh your memory,
Dr. Ringer's research and tests indicated that calcium
and potassium had counter-balancing effects which opposed one another in the regulation of the heart
rhythm and beat.

Potassium acted as a slowing agent—calcium to
speed and increase the vigor of the stroke. This discovery brought about the advent of electrolyte therapy,
which has been perhaps the greatest medical advance-
ment in modern history.

Today magnesium has been added to the formula, as
well as other minerals with electrolytic effects. But the
fact still remains that whether these minerals are inject-
ed into the bloodstream with a needle or taken in as
food in the diet, the basic physiological and nutritional
effect is the same.

Only the expediency of a heroic situation makes the
bloodstream method of introduction necessary. In fact,
potassium is preferably given by mouth to be absorbed
in the intestinal tract as there are certain risks involved
with the intravenous injection route.

Why has it been so difficult to study the physiological effects of minerals (which is the reason investigation has lagged)? The explanation is simple: While it is
comparatively easy to provide test animals with diets
lacking in a specific vitamin and so study the effect, it
is virtually impossible to feed the animals on a diet
which is free of a specific mineral. This is because
minerals are used in the body in comparatively large
amounts, while only infinitesimal amounts of vitamins
are required. Remember our example of only one milligram of vitamin B-1 as the minimum daily requirement,

compared to about 750 milligrams for calcium—and
about 1,500 milligrams estimated for potassium.

Now you understand why, when you supplement
your diet with minerals in tablet form, it is usually
necessary to consume a larger number of tablets than is
required for vitamins.

It is frequently a problem to the clinician when patients object to taking 12 or 14 mineral tablets per
day: how to overcome this objection? Simply by explaining that it is utterly impossible to concentrate
minerals any more than in the amounts nature provided them and, because large amounts are needed, a
greater number of tablets must be taken. (It doesn't always work. Some people have a phobia about taking a
large number of tablets.)

There is another facet of the mineral picture that
needs to be considered. That is what happens to them
after they get into the bloodstream, and into the
process of assimilation. The mineral solutions in the
blood (while important for ionic equilibrium—the balance between positive [acid] and negative [alkaline]
ions) serve no further purpose until they cross the cell
membrane and take part in the intercellular reactions.

It is within the cells themselves—not the bloodstream—that minerals perform their most important
work, both structurally and functionally. That is where
vitamins come into the picture. To mention a few effects of vitamins in mineral metabolism:
Vitamin D puts calcium to work in the cells as a structural element.
Vitamin B-6 helps potassium across the cell membranes.
Vitamins A and C metabolize calcium in the formation
of tooth structures.

Another consideration in mineral metabolism is their

interrelated effects. Phosphorus and calcium counterbalance one another; potassium and sodium do the same. The potassium-sodium ratio is particularly important as sodium is one mineral of which we can get too much. This "pushes" potassium out of the tissue storehouses and it is excreted in the urine. Up to nine times as much potassium may be excreted by persons eating all the ordinary table salt they want as compared with those on a salt-restricted diet.

What is the best way to assure an ample supply of minerals in the diet? Plenty of fresh vegetables and dairy products (such as raw milk, yogurt and natural cheeses) is the answer. But do not throw that cooking water away (nor fluid from canned vegetables either). About a third of the minerals are in the fluid or juice. That's a pretty high proportion, isn't it? Remember this about minerals: They work in unison and are interrelated in their nutritional effects. Like vitamins, only a complete pattern of the various mineral complexes is sufficient to do the job.

Pay more attention to the minerals in your diet— even if you can't find a textbook telling you exactly why. The experience and good health of multitudes of believers should be enough to convince you of the necessity for an adequate and balanced supply.

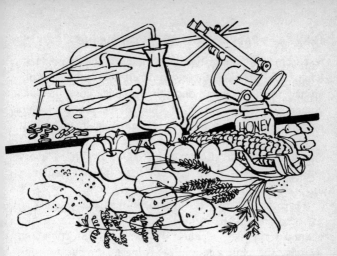

Chapter VII

ORGANIC OR SYNTHETIC?

THERE IS much confusion regarding the efficacy of the cheaper, synthetic varieties of food supplements flooding the market today. The controversy should help nutritional novices who have mistakenly purchased a synthetic product under the assumption that it was organic because it was purchased in a health food store. It is an unfortunate fact of life that many people demand and insist upon high-potency products. Because of this, the health food store proprietor is literally forced to stock and make available such items in order to satisfy his clientele and remain a profit-making business in the free enterprise tradition. The mistaken concept that high potency is equivalent to high activity is a direct result of the advertising campaigns of large chemical suppliers selfishly creating the impression and misconception that potency equals quality. Independent research and exhaustive experimentation have challenged and rebuked these unproven claims but the obviously misleading and deceptive practice continues unabated. A direct result of this mercenary onslaught against millions and millions of more health-conscious Americans than ever is the oft-heard wail of the disenchanted synthetic vitamin user: "Oh, I've tried every kind of vitamins there are but they haven't helped a bit."

There is certainly no argument that the chemist in his laboratory can produce what he considers perfect chemical replicas of natural vitamins. Unfortunately, we have the same condition existing as the curator who did not have a supply of real sea water for his ocean fish. His chemist assured the troubled curator that this presented no serious problem as the chemical composition of sea water was well known and he could easily create an ample supply. But almost as soon as the ocean fish were introduced into the chemical "sea" water they suffered and died. The chemist, believing only that he had probably erred in his composition made another batch with even more careful attention to detail and proportions. A second school of fish suffered the same fate; subsequent batches also failed to survive. Then another curator with a somewhat better supply of common sense added minute parts of real sea water to the artificial concoction and the fish lived happily ever after.

Even in the face of evidence of this conclusive nature, a majority of chemists today still will not accept a difference between synthetically manufactured vitamins and those derived from natural food sources. Such stubborn adherence to unsubstantiated and unproven theory is a true stumbling block to proper clinical evaluation of food concentrate, vitamin complex, mineral complex or whatever. For example, one research group uses a substance derived from natural food sources and notes the response in many different patients, thus eliminating the variables; the group then publishes its findings in a professional journal encouraging another laboratory to duplicate the experiment. A second group obeys every rule of research using identical environment, diet and controls, but fails to question the source of the substance under surveillance because it was tagged with a name such as "vitamin M." Now, the second group has as its source of supply a local pharmaceutical house which uses a synthetic version of group one's natural vitamin "M." The results of this test may be completely different from the original because of the lack of some unknown substance, as yet unidentified, which is present in an organic complex but not in a chemical complex. Variations in sources, such as exemplified in the foregoing, have to a great extent contributed to the loud and continuing squabble over the effectiveness of supplementation as a means of therapy.

Without equivocation, products made from chemicals will never compare favorably with the products of nature. The living cell of the plant is a complex compilation of life-giving rays of the sun, minerals derived from fertile soil, vitamins, enzymes, amino acids and the many unknown substances which make up life. It is important to clarify the little-known difference between a synthetic, a crystalline and a natural vitamin. The synthetic is obviously just what it says—the end product of a chemist's compilation from inorganic substances. Such products are sold at cut-rate prices because their source material is readily available and cheap, usually coal tar or other petroleum derivatives. A crystalline vitamin is a natural substance subjected to various means of processing in order to get a single substance in concentration. The end product is a highly refined, concentrated, crystalline substance without any contamination of the elements with which it was originally associated. This product is usually sold under the banner "From natural sources." The discerning health-conscious buyer will note that the high-potency contents listed on the label are never found in nature. On the other hand, a completely natural vitamin is of necessity low potency, but does contain the synergistic substances naturally contained in an organic combination. A compromise has taken place in the field of tablet making, where the crystalline vitamins are put in a natural base thus achieving the benefits of both—high potency and synergistic activity.

I am unalterably opposed to using single high-potency substances indiscriminately. A good reason for not taking highly purified single substances is the imbalance which the excess intake of a single vitamin factor may produce. Vitamin B-1 is an excellent example of this. We know that without adequate amounts of vitamin B-6 in the system, the excess B-1 may produce a deficiency of B-6 with resultant severe symptoms. Vitamins are associated together in nature and work together in our bodies—it is folly to take isolated, high-potency substances and expect to receive benefits. Incidentally, vitamin E is another good example of this. A large intake of vitamin E should always be balanced with adequate calcium as this is a synergistic necessity for vitamin E utilization.

It behooves everyone interested in regaining or maintaining health to distinguish which is more important and makes more sense: a one-sided, unbalanced, enzyme deficient, synergistic deficient, synthetic, high-potency vitamin, or a natural food complex containing the balances of ingredients as found in nature. The answer is—or should be—naturally obvious.

HOW TO KNOW IF VITAMINS ARE HELPING

One of the most disturbing remarks a nutritionist can hear is said when he is explaining what symptoms a vitamin might correct and the person being interviewed interjects with the remark, "I don't have that . . ." On the surface, the remark seems innocent enough, but to the person conducting the interview it shows clearly that the listener does not understand the basic principles involved in nutritional supplementation.

When the nutritional effects of vitamins are given, each is characterized by a list of symptoms that they have been shown to correct. Vitamin B-6, for example, may correct symptoms such as muscle cramps, numbness, insomnia, fluid retention and tremors when nutritionally caused. Persons who have one or more of these symptoms, who are deficient in vitamin B-6, may get relief from its use. But this symptomatic relief is the smallest part of the matter. Symptoms are, in fact, only the top of the iceberg whose main bulk remains hidden in the biological waters beneath the surface.

It is not nearly so important that this or that symptom be corrected—however dramatic the result may be—as the fact that all attending symptoms related to the vitamin's physiological effects may be prevented. A much better attitude than "I don't have that . . ." would be "I don't want to get that . . ." That's where really sound judgment in nutritional considerations begins.

Another point of concern for nutritionists is when the person being interviewed remarks, "I'll take it for a few days and see if it helps me." The snag in that statement is "see if it helps me." (The "few days" part I do not mind.) The fact is that unless the person knows what to look for, he may be greatly helped without the knowledge that it is helping him at all.

The classical example of this type of incident was a kindly lady to whom I had recommended a vitamin on the basis of a well-defined group of symptoms which she said were bothering her. About a week later she was contacted again. The conversation went something like this: "Are you taking the vitamin I recommended?" "Haven't missed a day." "Are you still bothered with falling asleep?" "Not lately." "How about letting dishes fall when you're at work?" (She was employed as a waitress.) "Didn't let any fall this week." "Have the muscle cramps cleared up?" "Completely." "Then you must be feeling better?" "No, as a matter of fact, I don't feel any better at all."

Such a confused attitude is more common than you may think. There are many symptoms which clear up when taking vitamins of which the user may be completely unaware because he never attributed them to a vitamin deficiency in the first place.

It is very difficult, for example, to get a person with a chronic back pain to admit that his problem may have its roots in nutritional causes. If given a supplement that relaxes the muscles that are attached to the spine, thus relieving intervertebral pressure, he is very likely to conclude that he is having one of his good spells and never relate the relief to the supplement he may be taking.

The same type of misconception can often apply to headaches, "nervous" stomach, insomnia, rheumatism and a host of other discomforting complaints. It is not that these are vague symptoms, but rather that because they may be transient in nature the consumer of vitamins never relates their relief to the food supplements he is taking.

The lesson to be learned here is that you have to become a proficient observer of the relationship between cause and effect to really learn whether vitamins are helping you. Just feeling better or worse is not enough reason to take or not to take vitamins; you need to learn what is being corrected, then continue its use to prevent its re-occurrence when nutritional deficiencies are the cause.

Such inconsistencies between fact and fancy are one of the main obstacles to a wider application of nutritional supplementation than is being applied today. But, you say, "I'm not a doctor; how can I know what's going on in my body?" That does not make sense either. You must remember that most of the symptoms caused by nutritional deficiencies are of the subjective variety. Subjective symptoms are the type which are only known to the patient, like headaches, cramps, insomnia, nervousness, indigestion and so forth. Your doctor would never know that they existed if you did not tell him.

It is true that their significance can better be interpreted by a doctor, but the fact remains that recognition of their existence is only made by you. So, as an individual trying to learn whether vitamins are helping you or not, you need to place a strong emphasis on subjective symptoms in relationship to the food supplements you are taking. Write them down one by one and check back on your list after taking vitamins for a reasonable period of time. You may be surprised at what you learn.

We have often heard persons say, "I wouldn't be without my vitamin E or vitamin C." It is obvious that they have taken them and achieved results they can feel. But often these same persons show a disregard of the many other nutritional factors which could be of benefit to their health. A good multiple vitamin and mineral supplement may add immeasurably to improving the nutritional patterns of their diets.

There is no experiment so fascinating as one in which you are personally involved. The nutritional experiment—and it is an experiment—is as personal as any in the world. But experimentation in this respect is not to be regarded as using yourself as a guinea pig. Far from it. You are really experimenting (if that is the word) with a scientifically established biochemical factor (vitamins) to determine its benefits to you as an individual—what it will do for you as a person, how you yourself are involved. It is like the mechanic who experiments to find the trouble with your car. He may install a new generator and fail to correct what is wrong. True, he didn't correct the problem, but he did no harm. Again, he may diagnose the problem as a faulty thermostat and hit the nail on the head; all is well and the motor does not heat up. That is the type of experimenting that you do when you are trying to find out whether vitamins are helping you or not.

It is becoming more evident all the time that this type of personal experimentation is being frowned upon by certain factions in orthodox fields. That is not bad; it is good. But instead of attempting to suppress this honest effort on the part of health-conscious persons, they should be providing guidelines for them to follow.

No such information has been forthcoming and probably never will be. This leaves us right where we started. There is only one way to know if the vitamins you are taking are helping you and that is by common sense evaluations made by yourself. It is a matter of trying the shoes on to get one that fits. At least that is what we have to work with at the present time.

VITAMIN AND MINERAL GUIDE

It is necessary for the body to maintain a balance of vitamins and minerals in the system to provide a full and healthy life. Deficiencies of these natural life-giving elements in various degrees often result in certain commonly accepted ailments under specified conditions. For this reason, the following Vitamin and Mineral Guide has been included in this work. The symptoms noted herein, of course, could occur only when the daily intake of the vitamins or minerals mentioned have been less than the minimum daily requirement over a prolonged period of time. These non-specific symptoms do not alone prove a nutritional deficiency but may be caused by any great number of conditions or functional causes. If such symptoms persist, a condition other than a vitamin or mineral deficiency could be indicated and competent, professional help should immediately be sought.

VITAMIN A

Also known as the anti-infective or anti-ophthalmic vitamin. Usually measured in USP (United States Pharmacopeia) Units. Natural sources are fruits and vegetables, dairy products, eggs, greens, fish liver oils, liver, etc. Builds resistance to infections, especially of the respiratory tract. Helps maintain a healthy condition of the outer layers of many tissues and organs. Permits formation of visual purple in the eye, counteracting night blindness and weak eyesight. Promotes growth, vitality and a healthy skin; essential for pregnancy and lactation. A deficiency may result in night blindness, increased susceptibility to infections, dry and scaly skin, lack of appetite and vigor, defective teeth and gums and retarded growth.

VITAMIN B-1

Thiamine, Thiamine Chloride; also known as the anti-neuritic or anti-beriberi vitamin. Measured in milligrams (mg). Natural sources are dried yeast, rice husks, whole wheat, oatmeal, peanuts, most vegetables, milk, etc. Promotes and aids growth and digestion; essential for normal functioning of nerve tissues, muscles and heart. Deficiencies may lead to loss of appetite, weakness and lassitude, nervous irritability, insomnia, loss of weight, vague aches and pains, mental depression and constipation. Deficiency in children may cause impaired growth.

VITAMIN B-2

Riboflavin or vitamin G; measured in milligrams (mg). Natural sources are liver, kidney, milk, yeast, cheese and most B-1 sources. Improves growth, promotes general health and is essential for healthy eyes, skin and mouth. Deficiency may result in itching and burning of the eyes, cracking of the corners of the lips, inflammation of the mouth, bloodshot eyes, purplish tongue.

VITAMIN B-6

Pyridoxine; measured in milligrams (mg). If designated in micrograms (mcg), remember that it requires 1000 micrograms to equal 1.0 milligram (mg). Natural sources are meat, fish, wheat germ, egg yolk, cantaloupe, cabbage, milk, yeast, etc. Aids in food assimilation and in protein and fat metabolism; prevents nausea and various nervous and skin disorders. A deficiency may result in nervousness, insomnia, skin eruptions, loss of muscular control.

VITAMIN B-12

Commonly known as the "red vitamin" cobalamin. Since it is so effective in small dosages, it is the only common vitamin generally expressed in micrograms (mcg). Found naturally in liver, beef, pork, eggs, milk, cheese, etc. Helps in the formation and regeneration of red blood cells thus helping prevent anemia; promotes growth and increased appetite in children; a general tonic for adults. Deficiency may lead to nutritional and pernicious anemia, tiredness, poor appetite and growth failure in children.

VITAMIN C

Ascorbic acid, cevitamic acid; expressed in milligrams (mgs), occasionally in Units. 1.0 mg equals 20 Units. Found naturally in citrus fruits, berries, greens, cabbages, peppers. (Easily destroyed by cooking.) Vitamin C is necessary for healthy teeth, gums and bones; strengthens all connective tissue; promotes wound healing; helps promote capillary integrity and prevention of permeability; an important factor in maintaining sound health and vigor. Deficiencies may lead to soft gums, tooth decay, loss of appetite, muscular weakness, skin hemorrhages, capillary weakness, anemia.

VITAMIN D

Viosterol, ergosterol; "sunshine" vitamin." Measured in USP Units. Natural sources are fish-liver oils, fat, eggs, milk, butter, sunshine, etc. Regulates the use of calcium and phosphorus in the body and is therefore necessary for the proper formation of teeth and bones. Very important in infancy and childhood. Deficiency may lead to rickets, tooth decay, retarded growth, lack of vigor, muscular weakness.

VITAMIN E

Tocopherol; available in several different forms and generally designated according to its biological activity in International Units (IU). Found naturally in wheat germ oil, whole wheat, green leaves, vegetable oils, meat, eggs, whole grain cereals, etc. The exact functions of vitamin E in humans are not yet known. Medical articles have been published on its value in helping to prevent sterility; in the treatment of threatened abortion; in muscular dystrophy; prevention of deposits in blood vessel walls. Has also been used favorably by some doctors in the treatment of heart conditions. Has wide public acceptance in the treatment of burns, cuts and bruises and as an aid to a vibrant and healthy skin and complexion. A deficiency may lead to increased fragility of red blood cells. In experimental animals, deficiencies led to loss of reproductive powers and muscular disorders.

VITAMIN F

Unsaturated fatty acids, linoleic acid and linolenic acids. Found naturally in vegetable oils such as soybean, peanut, safflower, cottonseed, corn and flaxseed. Necesssary for healthy skin, hair and glands; a growth-promoting factor. Promotes the availability of calcium to the cells; considered to be important in lowering blood cholesterol and in combatting heart disease. A deficiency may lead to skin disorders such as eczema.

VITAMIN K

Menadione. Natural sources are alfalfa and other green plants, soybean oil, egg yolks, etc. Vitamin K is essential for the production of prothrombin (a substance which aids the blood in clotting) and is important to normal liver function. Deficiency may lead to hemorrhages resulting from prolonged blood-clotting time.

VITAMIN P

Citrus bioflavonoids, bioflavonoid complex, hesperidin. Natural sources are citrus fruit peels and pulp, especially lemons. Strengthens the walls of capillaries; prevents vitamin C from being destroyed in the body by oxidation; beneficial in hypertension; helps build resistance to infections and colds. A deficiency may lead to capillary fragility or an appearance of purplish spots on the skin.

NICOTINIC ACID (Niacin); NIACINAMIDE
(Nicotinamide)

The functions and deficiency symptoms of these members of the B complex are similar. Niacinamide is more generally used since it minimizes the burning, flushing and itching of the skin that frequently occurs when using nicotinic acid. Found naturally in liver, lean meat, whole wheat products, yeast, green vegetables, beans, etc. Important for the proper functioning of the nervous system; prevents pellagra; promotes growth; maintains normal function of the gastrointestinal tract. Necessary for metabolism of sugar and to maintain normal skin conditions. A deficiency may result in pellagra, symptoms of which include inflammation of the skin and tongue; also gastrointestinal disturbance, nervous system dysfunction, headaches, fatigue, mental depression, vague aches and pains, irritability, loss of appetite, neuritis, loss of weight, insomnia, general weakness.

CALCIUM PANTOTHENATE

Pantothenic acid; a member of the B-complex family. Found naturally in liver, kidney, yeast, wheat, bran, peas, crude molasses. Calcium pantothenate functions are not yet clearly defined. Helps in the building of body cells and maintaining normal skin, growth and development of the central nervous system. Required for synthesis of antibodies; necessary for normal digestive processes. Originally believed to be a factor in restoring gray hair to original color but this function has not been substantiated. A deficiency may lead to skin abnormalities, retarded growth, painful and burning feet, dizzy spells, digestive disturbances.

FOLIC ACID

A member of the vitamin B complex. Natural sources are deep green, leafy vegetables, liver, kidney, yeast, etc. Essential to the formation of red blood cells by its action on the bone marrow. Aids in protein metabolism and contributes to normal growth. A deficiency may result in nutritional macrocytic anemia.

CHOLINE

A member of the B-complex family; one of the "lipotropic factors." Found naturally in egg yolks, brain, heart, green leafy vegetables and legumes, yeast, liver and wheat germ. Regulates function of the liver; necessary for normal fat metabolism; minimizes excessive deposits of fat in liver. A deficiency may result in cirrhosis and fatty degeneration of the liver and hardening of the arteries.

INOSITOL

Another member of the B-complex family. Natural sources are fruits, nuts, whole grains, milk, meat, yeast, etc. Inositol's functions and deficiency factors are similar to those of choline.

METHIONINE

One of the essential amino acids. Found naturally in meat, eggs, fish, milk, cheese, etc. Builds new body tissue; helps to remove fat from liver. Deficiency may lead to fatty degeneration and cirrhosis of the liver.

BIOTIN

One of the latest members of the B-complex family to be discovered. Natural source is yeast; present in minute quantities in every living cell. Biotin is a growth-promoting factor; possibly related to metabolism of fats and to the conversion of certain amino acids. A deficiency may lead to extreme exhaustion, drowsiness, muscle pains and loss of appetite; also could result in a type of anemia complicated by a skin disease.

LYSINE

L-lysine monohydrochloride; one of the essential amino acids. Found naturally in meat, eggs, fish, milk, cheese, etc. Builds new body tissue and vital substances such as antibodies, hormones, enzymes and body cells. Deficiency factors are not yet definitely known.

RUTIN

The natural source of rutin is buckwheat. Functions are similar to those of vitamin P: strengthens walls of capillaries; prevents vitamin C from being destroyed in body by oxidation; beneficial in hypertension and possibly helps build resistance to infections and colds. A deficiency can lead to capillary fragility and the appearance of purplish spots on the skin much as in a deficiency of vitamin P.

PABA

Para-amino-benzoic acid; belongs to the B-complex group. The natural source of PABA is yeast and it functions as a growth-promoting factor, possibly in conjunction with folic acid. When omitted from foods in experimental tests on animals, the lack of this vitamin caused hair to turn white. When restored to the diet, the white hair turned black. A deficiency may cause extreme fatigue, eczema, anemia.

THE IMPORTANT MINERALS

CALCIUM

Builds and maintains bones and teeth; helps blood to clot; aids vitality and endurance; regulates heart rhythm.

COBALT

Stimulant to production of red blood cells; component of vitamin B-12; necessary for normal growth and appetite.

COPPER

Necessary for absorption and utilization of iron, formation of red blood cells.

FLUORINE

Acts with calcium to strengthen bones and teeth.

IODINE

Necessary for proper function of thyroid gland; essential for proper growth, energy and metabolism.

IRON

Required in manufacture of hemoglobin; helps carry oxygen in the blood.

MAGNESIUM

Necessary for calcium and vitamin C metabolism; essential for normal functioning of nervous and muscular system.

MANGANESE

Activates various enzymes and other minerals; related to proper utilization of vitamins B-1 and E.

MOLYBDENUM

Associated with carbohydrate metabolism.

PHOSPHORUS

Needed for normal bone and tooth structure; interrelated with action of calcium and vitamin D.

POTASSIUM

Necessary for normal muscle tone, nerves, heart action and enzyme reactions.

SULPHUR

Vital to healthy skin, hair and nails.

ZINC

Helps normal tissue function, protein and carbohydrate metabolism.

PROTEIN FACTS

It is very easy, indeed, to find ourselves consuming vast, unnecessary quantities of calories to get the other essential foodstuffs we need. The researches of recent years have shown that most of us get too much of the nonperishable and nonessential factors and too little of the organic minerals and vitamins.

Another question arises: Do we get enough amino acids from the protein we eat?

POTATO PROTEIN BEST

Maybe we get enough protein—in all probability, too much—but it may be of such low grade that we will suffer from a deficiency of amino acids.

What are the major sources of protein? It may be surprising to some to learn that a scientist from Denmark concluded that potato protein was the best of all proteins for human nutrition. But, since potato solids are only 10 percent protein, we say we cannot tolerate the starch. We forget that potato starch has an alkaline ash, and is far better tolerated than the acid ash starch of the cereals. Actually, if we supplement potatoes with meat or beans, we arrive at a pretty good diet. The vegetarian can supplement his potatoes with raw milk, cheese, beans and bean sprouts.

Most meat is just muscle. The rare amino acids needed to protect, repair or build the glandular organs must come from similar glandular organs, from the liver, kidney, pancreas or sweetbreads. And we should not forget skin and what is commonly referred to as tripe, as both also contain rare amino acids.

REASONS FOR ALLERGIES

For protein to be absorbed it must be split into

amino acids so that it can penetrate the membranous walls of the alimentary tube; for proteins, as such, are not diffusible through the membranous tissue. If proteins do pass through without first being completely broken down, they may cause allergic reactions. A rather well accepted theory of allergic disease is that it results from a weakness in the pancreas. This causes weaker proteolytic enzymes which are not able to complete their tasks of breaking down the proteins into the amino acids. These incompletely broken down proteins can, in the presence of colitis or other irritated states of the intestinal tract, get into the general circulation. The immunity mechanism reacts immediately; from that time on it is possible that you will have an allergy to whatever type of protein you were eating at that particular time. This situation may also occur when you have overeaten a certain food, or even many foods, and the digestive system has not been able to handle the whole completely.

We must also remember that a lack of digestive factors, such as hydrochloric acid, will also produce effects similar to those noted above. The first stage in the digestion of a protein includes the need for hydrochloric acid.

Thousands of years ago the Chinese invented an amino acid product which we now refer to as soy sauce. This is made by hydrolyzing vegetable proteins with enzymes and preserving the resulting liquid with salt.

TEMPERAMENTAL AMINO ACIDS

Amino acids are temperamental and easily destroyed by heat. It is for this reason that the meat you eat should be rare, never well-done. (You will avoid pork entirely. See Chapter II .) Research has even demonstrated that in the case of animals (dogs), a diet of well-done meat is more detrimental than a starvation diet. This should cause some of us considerable concern when we decide on our foods for table consumption.

LIVER IMPORTANT

It is important to remember that protein metabolism is dependent upon liver integrity; factors that embarrass the liver interfere with protein metabolism and may result in nutritional deficiency. The liver is very frequently abused by the excess use of vitamin B-1 by well-meaning individuals. Cirrhosis and degenerative changes result if the rest of the B complex is not supplied in sufficient quantity. This toxic reaction is more common than most people realize. Many individuals report that certain vitamin B preparations (usually synthetic) which they have used created unfavorable reactions. These are usually corrected by treatment directed to the liver.

I definitely do not wish to leave the impression that vitamin B supplementation is not good. On the contrary, I highly recommend it, but always specify that the complete B complex be used, not single factors.

A deficiency of phosphorus has also been demonstrated to be inhibitory to liver function. A very simple way of adding this substance to the diet is via lecithin.

WISE NATIVES

Every month, research is demonstrating that amino acids are important for our well-being. In fact, it is now admitted that ingesting the specialized amino acids of brain tissue will enhance the ability of one's brain to restore and rebuild itself. This is also true of other organs; now we can scientifically prove it but the natives knew it long before the advent of civilization. When they wanted more stamina, better health, etc., they always ate raw, fresh organ meat.

Let us consider the largest group of chronically ill persons in the United States today—the heart patients. They are ideal prospects for amino acid supplementation and treatment. The degeneration which has set in during years of abuse can be better repaired if the essential building blocks are present. Often the greatest impediment in these cases is the lack of tools the body needs to repair itself. This of course includes the growth vitamins and their partners, the amino acids. Amazingly enough, ulcer patients and persons suffering from a host of seemingly unrelated disorders also respond quite rapidly when the raw materials are present.

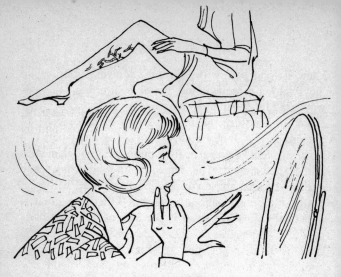

Chapter VIII

FOR WOMEN ONLY

BEAUTY AND YOUR HEALTH

EVERY TIME you see a person with healthy skin and hair, there is an attractiveness that cannot be denied. On the other hand, when unhealthy skin and hair are observed, even the most striking physical appearance suffers a disadvantage in esthetic appeal. Every race marks its classical beauties by their complexions. Doctors are not exempt.

An appraisal of the health of the skin and hair is an important consideration in every routine physical examination. These so-called cosmetic effects are, then, valued not only for the glamor they add to your personality, but for hygienic reasons as well.

Of course, skin and hair health begins with the diet. However, while vitamin A has been given most of the credit as the skin vitamin, our experience shows that the skin mineral potassium is much more effective in correcting nutritional deficiencies more directly concerned with many common skin problems, such as acne, dry skin, skin which is tender and easily chafed and irritated, even many so-called "allergic" reactions causing the skin to be highly sensitive to chemical agents.

I have observed, however, that not every potassium will do the job equally well. It is the inorganic salt of potassium (potassium chloride) which is the most effective nutritional form. This is the same potassium salt found in the modified salt mentioned in Chapter III. Potassium chloride is also available in supplemental tablet form as a food for special dietary use. The diet should be relatively free of refined sugar as well, for best results.

The skin needs the same natural care from the outside of the body as it does internally. Enhancing natural skin exfoliation is the best way of providing this care.

This is because the skin is constantly shedding the cells of its lifeless outer layer, which acts as a mask for new cells arising underneath. The faster this masking layer is removed, the fresher and healthier will be the appearance of the skin and hair—like the soft, moist skin after peeling from suntanning.

Physiologists estimate that we have a completely new skin every two to three weeks by the normal shedding process. In expensive beauty emporiums, this process is hastened by a process known as skin scraping, which can be painful, time-consuming and costly—although admittedly effective.

That is the hard way! The easy, natural way to unmask the skin, removing the lifeless outer layer, is by the use of colloidal gel suspension of translucent beneficiated clay. This unique natural mineral substance has the rare physical property of causing lifeless protein molecules (of which the outer skin surface is composed) to adhere to themselves, acting like a "molecular sponge" to cleanse and rid the skin, hair and scalp of extraneous materials. (Unlike ordinary clays, beneficiated clay is predominantly a magnesium compound as opposed to the usual aluminum silicate comprising the common gray, brown or bluish clays usually used for cosmetic purposes, such as in clay packs.)

Unlike soaps and detergents, which have a chemical, solvent-type action, beneficiated clay is entirely mechanical in the way it works, lifting or "sweeping" away lifeless cells and debris with a cleansing action for natural exfoliation.

Technically, this is called adsorption. It is useful to think of the action of beneficiated clay in the same manner as one does the action of cultivating in organic farming. The natural look of the skin is developed, without artificial means, so that the pores are left in their virgin state, free of substances which might clog or otherwise inhibit their normal function. The slightly acid pH of the skin and scalp remains unchanged (alkaline soaps and detergents alter this natural environment).

Lest you have been led to believe this method is something new, let us assure you it is not. The well-known mud baths of the Greeks and Romans, famed for their beautifying effects, were, no doubt, the practical application of the method we have been describing. It could well have been one of Cleopatra's secrets, brought to you by Egyptian cosmetologists who discovered such a sedimentary deposit along the banks of the

Nile or its delta. Her diet, rich in fresh fruits, grapes, pomegranates and dates was, undoubtedly, rich in potassium as well. Legend aside, of such things are healthy, beautiful skin and hair made.

It is really quite easy to apply these natural cosmetic principles in our modern times. The diet should be high in vegetables, proteins and bulk-producing foods to promote normal elimination. Substitute the new modified salt for the ordinary salt you may be using. Keep refined sugars off the menu entirely, or at least use them with extreme moderation. Supplement the diet with a good all-around natural supplement, including vitamin A, as well as a well balanced mineral supplement which provides a daily intake of from one to one and one-half grams (1 gram is 1000 milligrams) of potassium chloride along with calcium, iodine and other ionizable minerals. Use beneficiated clay for all body and hand cleansing purposes, eliminating irritating soap and detergent products entirely.

Do this for only two weeks and you should have every right to expect a marked improvement in the health of your skin, hair and scalp, as well as experiencing other material benefits to your health by the improvement in balance of your body chemistry.

One skin problem about which we have particular concern is the acne confronting so many of our children. This occurs at a tender age, when such a marring affliction is apt to be a real psychological trauma. It is our conviction that the rapid cell growth of the "shooting up" period of life causes a vastly increased need for potassium, which is further aggravated by a diet high in salt and sugar characteristic of many foods teenagers seem to crave.

VARICOSE VEINS—INEVITABLE?

How many of you espoused men have received a well-placed elbow in your rib cage because you gazed a moment too long at a well-turned ankle?

Let us not try to fool ourselves; one of woman's greatest attributes is a well-shaped leg with pleasing, smooth contour. And yet, when we examine most women over thirty-five years of age, we see the beginning of ugly varicosities with their tortuous pathways interfering with the normal curves that are woman's heritage.

By no means should this be taken as an indication that women are the only victims. Men suffer almost as much as women do, but clothing covers their abnormalities—and man does not depend on his physical attributes as much as he does his pocketbook to lure the opposite sex.

The general attitude towards varicose veins is an unconcerned acceptance, with the idea that they are the natural, although troublesome, companions of middle and old age. When the pain becomes too severe, a stripping operation is performed in which the veins are removed. It should always be well remembered that the removal of veins for such reasons can usually be easily avoided by the proper use of diet, exercise and common sense. In addition, such stripping creates an increased demand upon other veins to carry the blood back to the heart and lungs.

POSTURE AS A FACTOR

The accumulated congestion in the lower extremities which is inherent in the upright posture of man can be considered as a definite factor in the gradual loss of tone in the venous system which may predispose one to varicose veins.

This situation can be alleviated by frequent and habitual use of the slant board or some other means of reversing the blood flow. The practice of standing on your head is excellent, although I advise using one of the many devices which are stabilizing aids in this exercise. Such simple procedures can add years of comfortable use to your legs and save you from the agony of swollen legs and strained blood vessels. Reversing the force of gravity appears to have a salutary effect on the blood flow to the entire body, and many have found that their mental acuity has been improved by these means.

FIENDISH INVENTION

The all too prevalent use of confining garments such as "extra slimming" girdles, etc., also plays a part in diverting nature's flow of life—the blood stream. Such fiendish inventions enable the female sex to misrepresent her attributes, and also allow her to slack off the exercise which is necessary to keep her shape and, more important, to keep her circulation active. These binding garments cut off circulation in the lower limbs. This sooner or later leads to stretching and breakdown of the veins, since they are superficial (nearest to the surface) and therefore affected more by binding, while the arteries keep pouring more blood into the extremities.

NUTRITIONAL AIDS

Nutritionally speaking, several vitamins and some other factors may be helpful in either prevention or relief. Part of the tone of the blood vascular system is dependent upon the body's receiving adequate rutin, a part of the vitamin C complex. It has been our custom to advise that the entire vitamin C complex be used with about 2000 milligrams of vitamin C, 400 milligrams of bioflavonoid complex and 200 milligrams of rutin. Vitamin E is important, and it has been my experience that the best results occur when an emulsified vitamin E complex is used at a rate of about 600 International Units per day.

The next most important factor involved is adequate liver function. I have never seen a case of varicose veins where there has not been a malfunctioning liver. The cleansing regimen for the liver, discussed in Chapter III, is certainly advocated and should be considered as a prerequisite for anyone with this problem. Once this has been carried out, enzymes and bile salts may be necessary to help the liver with some of its tasks. The herb collinsonia has been used for many years for assistance, and has withstood the test of time.

TOO SIMPLE?

Some who read the foregoing will say that I did not take into consideration the little valves in the veins which normally prevent the blood from flowing back and pooling in the vein. I sincerely believe that it is not the inability of these valves to function that creates the problem, but rather the stretching of the vein by excess back pressure, thus preventing the valve from doing an efficient job. Many have tried the regimen described here with excellent results. Remember, when you work with nature everything becomes simple.

THE MENOPAUSE AGE

At some time in every woman's life she must face the menopause. The tales of suffering and anguish can be heard at almost any gathering of the female sex. Several years ago a book was written extolling the virtues of estrogen to prevent the nerve-shattering symptoms which are suffered by some women during this difficult time of life.

It is now a common practice for practically every woman entering the menopause to receive either injectable or oral estrogen and often both. Is this a good practice? Are there any dangers? What are the advantages? Are there any alternatives? Let us go through these questions and determine if a logical answer can be reached.

As a brief review: the menopause is that time in a woman's life when her ovaries cease to function. Although all of the trials and problems that occur during the months or years before menstruation completely ceases and the time after such cessation are called menopause, this is technically incorrect. The true term is the climacteric, while menopause is only the stopping of menstrual activity. The climacteric is a period of transition during which a new endocrine equilibrium is established in which the ovaries have no part. Before this time they were actively secreting hormones which were in great part responsible for the female characteristics. The climacteric may commence months or even years before the final cessation of the ovarian function and extend just as long afterward. The amazing part to some women is that not every woman has the characteristic hot flashes, the weakness and prostration, the palpitating heart, the excessive perspiration, the dry mouth, the acute nervousness and personality changes, and a myriad other complaints. Some merely cease menstruating and that is it—no problems whatsoever.

MISCONCEPTIONS

One of the gravest misconceptions of the whole menopause is that at the time of cessation of menstruation all hormone output is stopped immediately. This is not true. There may be a reduction of these hormones but they are by no means just cut off. In order to illustrate this, let us bring to mind the woman who goes through the menopause without any symptoms whatsoever. The many changes which are supposed to take place in the female just do not happen. Why? Are these women abnormal or are all the others who have the symptoms the ones whose physiology is mixed up?

THE KEY

An often overlooked fact may be the key to understanding just what happens. Although the ovaries slowly or suddenly stop producing estrogen, the body is not slapped haphazardly together without any provision to substitute or take over function. At the time of the menopause the ovaries cease producing eggs and decrease their estrogen output, but adrenal and other glandular activity is stepped up to compensate for this loss. The adrenals being our glands of stress—the ones which prepare us for fight or flight—they are often already over-burdened today. There is evidence that the over-consumption of sugar has put a strain on these glands along with everything else. Now along comes the call to help take over the function of the ovaries. The already tired adrenal becomes more irritable and the following are the medical symptoms of adrenal irritability: dry mouth, circulatory imbalance (chills or flushing), temporary hypertension, internal nervousness and tremor, and abnormal perspiration. Do they sound familiar? Of course—they are the symptoms of the menopausal woman. The ovarian hormone along with potassium acts to inhibit the sympathetic nervous system. Without this inhibitor, sympatheticotonia may occur and blood which is normally pooled internally is suddenly rushed to the periphery which produces the hot flashes.

POTASSIUM AND VITAMIN E

It is interesting to note that potassium is an important mineral for proper adrenal function and also for controlling our sodium balance. To be completely in balance we should take in twice as much potassium as sodium in our daily diet. From all evidence which has been gathered, just exactly the opposite is true in the average diet—twice as much sodium as potassium. When sodium is overabundant, potassium is excreted out of the cell and lost through excretory mechanisms. Thus, we may get enough of this important mineral in our food but we have a sodium intake which is four times what it should be and the potassium is lost. Drugs such as the steroids and diuretics also force the excretion of this mineral. Because it is so necessary for glandular function, the menopause may be just the time for you to look to your potassium intake. Another factor which should be considered is vitamin E. Although not reported in glowing headlines, medical literature is full of articles by reputable researchers who have found that vitamin E is the most practical and effective treatment for menopausal symptoms including hot flashes, high blood pressure, nervousness, heart palpitations, shortness of breath, insomnia, dizziness, headaches, heavy menstrual flow, fatigue and others. What is the possible mechanism which makes vitamin E the key in these instances?

One should consider the original work done on wheat germ oil which indicated that there was a sex hormone precursor available in this substance. During the climacteric, when other endocrine glands are taking over the hormonal function of the ovaries, does it not make sense that a little spark in the form of a hormone precursor might be of great value?

For this reason, I always prefer a vitamin E which contains the raw wheat germ oil in addition to the alpha tocopherol. Many times it is the unknown substances which make the difference between success and failure. Many will wish to know how much to take and I can only generalize as research has indicated success at a wide range of dosage. My suggestion is 600 IU of d-alpha tocopherol, 1800 mg of raw wheat germ oil and 1800 mg of crude lecithin for emulsification purposes.

ESTROGEN THERAPY

The advent of estrogen therapy was one of the greatest symptom-relief therapies ever brought forth. Women on the brink of a nervous breakdown were miraculously brought back and became normal within a short time. I must say, however, that few miracles exist today. Every "miracle" drug which has been discovered is fraught with danger, too often a danger which is not readily apparent. We now hear almost daily reports (probably due to the investigation of birth control pills more than anything else) about the association of serious diseases with the use of estrogen therapy. I do not wish to give the impression that I am condemning estrogen therapy. I would never do so completely—but I cannot endorse it heartily. I feel that there are too many other possibilities for a woman to try to help her body adjust to a natural phenomenon. The use of estrogen may be necessary for short periods of time due to a physiological inability to adapt rapidly enough, but it should not be used as a crutch to stave off the inevitable.

HERBS ALSO VALUABLE

The natives of many lands do not have the modern laboratories to make drugs as we do and are forced to use nature as an assistant. Some of the herbs used through the ages for the climacteric are: Mexican damiana leaf, sarsaparilla root, cramp bark, squaw vine, and black haw bark. These are harmless and certainly are beneficial in a tonic sort of way and many women swear by them. By using common sense and assisting nature, I am sure that the menopause need hold no fear for you.

THE "INSTANT BREAKFAST" FRAUD

In our convenience-oriented society a new craze has struck—the so-called "instant" breakfasts. The concept is great and I have no particular quarrel with the idea of a meal in a glass—providing that glass has something more than just powdered skim milk in it. The present plethora of products are just that, with corn syrup solids for sweetening, artificial flavors and colors, synthetic vitamins and sugar. For this mixture the consumer pays from 10 to 30 cents per ounce, depending upon the manufacturer. Retail price of the ingredients if purchased separately would be approximately 2 cents per ounce, plus the synthetic vitamins—which, in my opinion, have little if any value.

The tragedy is that a mother thinks she is doing her children a favor by serving this potion to them at breakfast.

Children like sweet-flavored beverages and induce mother to use this product by the very vigor with which they down it. This brings another aspect of today's life into focus. Little Mary and Johnnie "don't like" cooked cereals made with whole grains. Usually they don't care for these things because Dad and Mother don't eat them either and Mother doesn't really want to take the time to prepare them. We are not born with likes and dislikes. A baby will eat with gusto a completely unflavored mixture that fills his stomach and provides him with nourishment. Hawiian children are completely pleased with poi, a rather gooey mixture with little flavor. When Mother, Dad, Grandma, etc. say "I can't stand broccoli," the conditioning has been set in motion so that chances are the young member of the family will also develop an aversion to this food.

So many times I have heard the mother tell me about her child: "The only vegetables he [or she] eats are green beans, peas and corn." It is my firm belief that the most important duty the mother has to her child is that of training the eating habits, to develop a broad acceptance of foods. It is an insurance policy against disease and the groundwork for greater achievement in both mental and physical spheres of endeavor.

I am frustrated beyond limits by the parent who informs me that not enough time is available to train a child properly. Health is wealth, and a few minutes taken each day with the goal in mind of furnishing a few different varieties of vegetables prepared in a tempting manner may have a profound effect on the life of the child entrusted to your care.

Instead of "instant breakfasts," may I suggest the use of this blender concoction: 8 ounces of soy milk, 1 raw egg, 2 tablespoons of a good quality protein (no less than 80 percent protein on a finished product basis), 1 tablespoon of blackstrap molasses and/or 1 tablespoon tupelo honey. You will now have a breakfast furnishing you with at least 30 grams of protein, approximately 250 calories and an abundance of natural vitamins, enzymes and minerals. To top it off, it is more tasty than that artificially-flavored powdered milk.

I might add a word about the controversy which always arises when raw egg is mentioned. An anti-enzyme known as avidin is found in raw egg white. This is rendered inactive when subject to heat. On this basis, many feel that egg should not be eaten raw because the avidin interferes with the digestion of the protein. In my opinion this would be true if only the white of an egg were eaten, but the yolk of the egg contains biotin, which is the product destroyed by avidin; thus we may not get the biotin from the egg but the raw enzymes and protein are beneficial. Because of this, I see no reason why the addition of a raw egg to such a health drink would have any undue effect. On the contrary it would furnish much in the way of proteins and vitamins.

GRANDMA'S REMEDIES

Many years ago, I was privileged to know and observe the wisdom of an old Indian medicine man practicing his profession in a primitive area of Idaho. This accomplished and successful Indian herbalist used only herbs found in nature, which he carefully gathered and prepared himself. Almost every time I went to see him he would have a huge stainless steel container simmering on the stove. The aroma of herbs permeated the room and the gallon jugs into which he poured the finished product lined the wall.

I was forced to use much finesse in trying to inveigle him into revealing his secrets, as he was quite suspicious and cantankerous by nature. In fact, the first time

I met him I spent the first half hour convincing him that I was not an agent of the FDA. It was only after a mutual friend, Dory Detton, solemnly vouched for my character, that the old man finally consented to accept me as a kindred soul.

To get back to the major lesson I learned from this Indian herbalist—he said that to cure most of the ills of the modern white man, all that was really necessary was to give him a good laxative. How simple, and yet how indicative of one of the most prevalent ills of our time. It is difficult for any serious ailment to attack the human system when the bowels are open. The other favorite remedy of this herbalist was a liver-cleansing regimen, which has been of assistance to me ever since.

Now for some common ailments and the old, time-honored remedies which are still practical.

BOILS—These usually are indicative of toxic wastes in the body, but also are a signal of thyroid deficiency. Calcium and magnesium are always indicated, and I often use a complex product consisting of kelp, dulse, hydrolyzed fish proteins and other factors to supply synergistic material for the normal functioning of the thyroid. Potato poultices are also excellent as an immediate relief and a means of bringing the boil to a head. The potato, peeling and all, should be finely grated and a small pack applied directly on the boil. Cover with gauze and hold in place with tape. Change twice a day.

MOTION SICKNESS and SEASICKNESS—Abstinence from a heavy meal, particularly heavy meats, just before taking the trip, and a preparatory period of three days using a vitamin C complex containing 250 milligrams of vitamin C eight times a day can usually control even serious cases. I have personally seen this work several times.

ULCERS—It is beyond me where the research work

demonstrating the efficacy of cabbage juice in treating ulcers is buried. If the ulcer sufferer will drink the juice of a raw head of cabbage every day, relief will be quick and sure in not more than ten days, although longer use is advised for long-lasting results. Another time-honored remedy is fenugreek and comfrey tea. Our source tells us this should be used at the rate of at least three cups per day. Fifteen drops of pure extract of aloe vera taken three times a day has provided relief for many in these gastric irritations. It is, of course, understood by all that such measures alone, without refraining from smoking and consumption of alcohol and without eating a proper diet, would be inadequate at best.

HEMORRHOIDS—A disorder which is often miraculously relieved by cleansing the liver. Many herbs are particularly recommended for this: mandrake, chicory, black cohosh, red sage, quassia, golden seal. Collinsonia is also recommended for hemorrhoids. A more common name for collinsonia is "stone root." This appears to be helpful in strengthening the tone of the blood vessels.

PARASITES OR WORMS—Garlic taken by mouth and also used in a high enema is effective. Raw pumpkin seeds are also helpful. Quassia and red sage are worthy of consideration and have proven their worth in practice.

DIARRHEA—Two tablespoons of pure carob in heated milk or added to a custard is a practical and safe approach to this disturbance. Fifteen drops of essence of peppermint in 4 ounces of hot water, repeated every two hours until relief is obtained, may also be used.

NATURAL LAXATIVE FOR BABIES—Equal parts of butter and honey blended together, or equal parts of safflower oil and honey. Dosage is ½ to 1 teaspoonful, repeated as needed. This causes no griping, contains no harsh irritants and most of all, it tastes good. (Note: Kleiner's *Physiology* states that even a relatively small amount of mineral oil will remove all carotene present in the food eaten and cause a deficiency of vitamin A. Mineral oil should never be used in any way by humans.)

ARTHRITIS—Several rules apply here, but the following are basically good, and also simple: (1) Eat a raw potato every day. (2) Use 1 tablespoon of raw wheat germ oil three times a day. (3) Take 2 teaspoons of concentrated sea water every day.* (4) Eliminate citrus foods and pasteurized milk from the diet.

COLDS—Mix 10 drops of spirits of camphor in one pint hot water. Sip within twenty minutes. This helps open the pores of the skin allowing the toxins to be eliminated. Always use copious quantities of vitamin C complex—500 to 1000 milligrams per hour.

COUGH SYRUP—Mix 2 ounces apple cider vinegar, 2 ounces of honey and 2 ounces of safflower oil. This is both soothing and healthful. Some add cayenne pepper or the herb lobelia to this concoction.

GALLSTONES—Allow me to warn you that the following formula is capable of dislodging a gallstone and it may be too large to pass down the duct. Such an occurrence leaves the patient in acute distress which may be intolerable. (1) No food of solid nature for three days. (2) For two days drink 1 pint of organic apple juice every two hours for six doses and use a mild herbal laxative each evening. (3) First thing in the morning on the third day, drink 2 glasses of apple

*Available at health food stores. To avoid pollution, do not collect your own.

juice and follow with 4 ounces of olive oil. (4) If there are no results by four p.m., repeat the morning procedure. This may also be repeated next morning. Success is noted when small greenish pebbles are found in the stool.

The foregoing is but a brief glimpse into the natural world of home remedies. In almost every household the world over can be found time-tested and trusted recipes of relief often reverently referred to as "Grandma's remedies"; one more solid affirmation that it is truly "a woman's world."

Chapter IX

CHARTING A HEALTHY COURSE

It is literally impossible to outline a nutritionally sound program applicable to all people. Every individual is the recipient of good health or the victim of poor health depending on his personal habits, environment, social status and, of course, his body chemistry. No one program or method can be a guarantee in charting a healthy course.

The Health Quotient following is a step in the right direction. It is widely accepted and utilized by many in the healing arts as an additional means of correlating problems of different natures, by presenting a more detailed and composite picture of the body and any malfunctions as a whole. Many of the questions are not usually asked by a doctor during routine examinations;

therefore, the Health Quotient can become an extremely valuable tool in early discovery of possible interrelated problem areas in our own systems.

IMPORTANT INSTRUCTIONS

Chart yourself by using the following numerical scoring index:

1—If the symptoms are mild.
2—If the symptoms are moderate.
3—If the symptoms are severe.

Check only those symptoms which apply to your case; do not write "No" where answers do not apply.

A score of three or more in any one section is indicative of a serious enough problem to be concerned. If your total group score is 0—5, consider yourself comparatively healthy (and continue to do whatever you are doing; it seems to be working); 6—10 is average, which means there are areas in which you should try to improve; if you score above 11, there is every indication you probably need expert, professional help.

As indicated at the beginning of this chapter, the Health Quotient is not to be construed as any more than a guide in our everlasting search for longer life and better health; the test certainly does not apply to everyone, but it does offer a certain and invaluable criteria to anyone seeking to retain or achieve optimum good health. The questionnaire is divided into four groups. (1) Gastrointestinal Indications. (2) Functional Nervous Indications. (3) Metabolic Indications; and (4) Hormone and Enzyme Indications. Each group is composed of several sections. Remember, your score is only an indication of your health; when in doubt, always consult professional help immediately. Now, on to Group One!

GROUP ONE - GASTROINTESTINAL INDICATIONS

Section A

1. (   ) Distress from fats or greasy foods, such as nausea, dizziness, headaches, etc.
2. (   ) Distress from onions, cabbage, radishes, cucumbers (cause bloating, gas, etc.)
3. (   ) Stool appears yellow, clay-colored; foul odored; shows undigested foods
4. (   ) Skin is grayish, pasty, oily on nose and forehead
5. (   ) Bad breath, bad taste in mouth, body odor (including feet)
6. (   ) Long history of constipation

Section B

1. (   ) Indigestion occurs 2 to 3 hours after meals, fullness, bloating, soreness, etc.
2. (   ) Heavy, full, loggy feeling after eating heavy meat meal
3. (   ) Loss of former taste or craving for meat
4. (   ) Excessive lower bowel gas (flatulence)
5. (   ) History of constipation which alternates with diarrhea (bowels "too loose or tight")

Section C

1. (   ) Stomach pain occurs 5 or 6 hours after eating, usually at night, relieved by eating or drinking milk or cream
2. (   ) Above symptoms flare up in spring and fall of year (seasonal occurrence)
3. (   ) Have been told you have stomach ulcers

Section D

1. (   ) Diarrhea occurs without apparent cause, resistant to ordinary treatment

2. (　　) Roughage in diet aggravates diarrhea
3. (　　) Mucous shreds appear in stool
4. (　　) Have more than three bowel movements per day

Section E

1. (　　) Indigestion occurs immediately after eating
2. (　　) Indigestion is acute, comes on suddenly
3. (　　) Have difficulty belching, stomach cramps, colicky, "butterfly" sensations in stomach

---

GROUP TWO - FUNCTIONAL NERVOUS INDICATIONS

Section A

1. (　　) Eyes are sensitive to bright lights such as headlights, sunlight, wear sunglasses
2. (　　) Have tightness in throat, "lump," hurts when emotionally disturbed
3. (　　) Form gooseflesh easily, sweat without temperature rise (cold sweats)
4. (　　) Voice rises to high pitch or is "lost" during stress such as arguments, public appearances, etc.
5. (　　) Easily shaken up, easily startled, heart pounds hard from unexpected noise
6. (　　) Prefer being alone, uneasy when center of attention
7. (　　) Blood pressure fluctuates, has been too high on occasion

Section B

1. (　　) Do you tend to work off worries; something left undone causes you unusual concern
2. (　　) Do you avoid complaints, try to ignore discomforts and inconveniences

3. (   ) Have you had frequent or severe attacks of pneumonia, bronchitis, flu, sinusitis

4. (   ) Have you had allergies such as skin rash, dermatitis, hay fever, severe sneezing attacks, asthma or other allergy

5. (   ) Do emotional storms cause complete exhaustion, must go and lie down when under heavy stress

6. (   ) Do you have an unusual craving for salt

7. (   ) Does your skin take on a brownish color, brown spots on skin (often called liver spots)

Section C

1. (   ) Are you unable to hold your breath for 20 seconds (use second hand on watch)

2. (   ) Do you sigh and yawn frequently

3. (   ) Do you have a feeling of suffocation, open windows in closed room

4. (   ) Do you feel short of breath at times, even though not exercising

5. (   ) Feel breathless when under stress

6. (   ) People remark that you "breathe loudly"; are heard breathing in quiet room

---

GROUP THREE - METABOLIC INDICATIONS

Section A

1. (   ) Are your muscles stiff in morning, feel need to limber up; feel "creaky" after sitting still for period of time

2. (   ) Feel dizzy or nauseated in morning

3. (   ) Motion sickness when traveling, dizzy when changing up and down positions

4. (   ) Does your heart occasionally seem to "miss beats or turn flip-flops"
5. (   ) Are following symptoms worse at night: coughing, hoarseness, muscle cramps
6. (   ) Do you have sleeplessness, restlessness, failing memory, forgetfulness
7. (   ) Do you feel better in the afternoon, worse in morning hours

Section B

1. (   ) Do you "go to pieces" easily, dislike working under pressure or being "watched," cry easily
2. (   ) Gain weight, fail to lose on diets
3. (   ) Long history of chronic constipation
4. (   ) Skin is thick, wrinkly, puffy
5. (   ) Feel better mornings, worse afternoons
6. (   ) Difficulty concentrating, easily distracted
7. (   ) On outer third of eyebrows is the hair unusually thin or absent

Section C

1. (   ) Does your heart beat above 90 beats per minute when at complete bed rest
2. (   ) Does protruding tongue quiver (use mirror), hands shake, tremor (use paper)
3. (   ) Do you have a strong drive followed by exhaustion; repeats in cycles
4. (   ) Do you have strong, healthy teeth
5. (   ) Do you have a good appetite, but fail to gain weight in spite of food increases
6. (   ) Fine features, thin skin, thin hair
7. (   ) Is your behavior erratic, "flighty"
8. (   ) Do you have poor balance (close eyes and stand on one leg)

GROUP FOUR - HORMONE AND ENZYME INDICATIONS

1. (   ) Muscle weakness, weak grip, weak legs
2. (   ) Numbness or loss of sensation, limbs "fall asleep"
3. (   ) Night sweats; wake up frightened
4. (   ) Allow objects to fall from hands
5. (   ) Muscle cramps, worse at night
6. (   ) Have had albumin in urine, kidney trouble
7. (   ) Ankles swell in hot weather

GROUP 5 - CAPILLARY INDICATIONS

1. (   ) Bruise easily, "black and blue spots"
2. (   ) Feel drowsy, chronic fatigue
3. (   ) Cold hands and feet, use extra clothing, bedclothing, heat pads to keep warm
4. (   ) Short of breath when climbing stairs
5. (   ) Require extra amount of sleep
6. (   ) Feel better when resting; lowered endurance, low exercise tolerance

GROUP SIX - CARBOHYDRATE INDICATIONS

Section A

1. (   ) Nervousness; shaky feeling; headaches are relieved by eating sweets
2. (   ) Irritable if late for meal, miss meal; before breakfast feel irritable
3. (   ) Experience sudden strong craving for sweets, alcohol
4. (   ) Get hungry "five minutes after eating"
5. (   ) Often wake up at night feeling hungry

Section B

1. (   ) Night sweats; increased thirst

2. (   ) Chronic fatigue, lowered resistance
3. (   ) History of boils, leg sores; lesions take long time to heal
4. (   ) Overweight
5. (   ) Feel pickup from exercising
6. (   ) At one time was told had sugar in urine, diabetes
7. (   ) Member of family has diabetes
8. (   ) Crave sweets, but eating sweets does not relieve symptoms

MALE:

1. (   ) Difficulty urinating, starting, burning; getting up nights
2. (   ) Associate above with back or leg pains, constipation
3. (   ) Have been told you have prostate trouble
4. (   ) Have had prostate surgery
5. (   ) Loss or diminished sex drive

FEMALE:

1. (   ) Irregular or discomforting periods
2. (   ) Menopause symptoms (hot flashes, etc.)
3. (   ) Have you had a female operation
4. (   ) Loss or diminished sex drive
5. (   ) Before periods feel nervous, depressed
6. (   ) Unable to have children because of sterility (not age or operation)

Now that you have completed this questionnaire, you may wonder what the various symptoms could mean. My first advice is to try and find a nutritionally-oriented physician who would be aware of potassium, calcium, vitamin E, B-complex, or other deficiency symptoms. Secondly, a study of the contents of this book and others dealing with nutritional deficiency

symptoms will pretty much give you all the information
you need.

WEEKLY DIET APPRAISAL

It is vitally important to keep an accurate record of
all the items of food and drink you consume during
certain designated periods to evaluate properly the information garnered from your Health Quotient. It is
recommended that a notebook be utilized to record all
food and drink consumed during a seven-day period. I
suggest this notebook be carried on your person and
completed on the spot rather than relying on memory
at some later date. An accurate record will contribute
to the appraisal value of the Health Quotient. Remember, all food and drink should be noted. Start with
breakfast and continue through lunch and dinner with
particular attention to all drinks, snacks, etc. consumed
between meals. It's your health that counts—so count
everything you eat or drink during the seven-day charting period. Your Diet Appraisal notebook will be an
invaluable tool for your doctor if professional help or
guidance is indicated after charting a healthy course as
outlined in this chapter. It might also surprise you
when you see all the "junk" you may be eating!

EACH DAY

BREAKFAST_____

LUNCH_____

DINNER_____

_____

BETWEEN-MEALS, DRINKS, SNACKS, ETC.

Sample daily form for recording all food and drink consumed during your 7-day charting period.

A HEALTHY VOYAGE TO YOU ALL!

You are now near the end of the first part of your journey to good health and a happier life through Preventive Organic Medicine. The suggestions and advice offered in your Passport to Good Health are only applicable, of course, when validated as part and parcel of your everyday life. You must read-study-meditate—then earnestly and conscientiously invoke and apply the basic truths of nature and common sense. The results to you and your loved ones will be tremendously exciting and inspiring as well as interesting to behold.

Just imagine the joy and elation of a person who perhaps has suffered from arthritis for many years without letup. Suddenly, changes in his body take place and relief from his agony is realized after years of believing there was no relief to be had. What a feeling of freedom it must be—similar to that of a prisoner shackled and sentenced to a life term without possibility of parole who finds new hope in the form of loosening of his bonds and commutation of his sentence. Thank God—and nature—for deliverance from our ills and the many misfortunes we so often bring upon ourselves.

After implementing the various programs contained herein, you will discover new and rewarding vistas opening within your nutritional world. Your new-found well-being and attitudes will be contagious—you will bring new hope and encouragement to many of your kindred brethren. I promise your reward will be pleasant, invigorating and, most of all, soul-satisfying. Sail on—to good health and long life. God bless you!

GLOSSARY

Acid Chemical term designating any compound that can react with a base to form a salt. The hydrogen of the acid is replaced by a positive ion.

Acid-base balance A balance between foods which leave an acid ash and those which leave an alkaline ash in the body.

Acne A skin eruption usually appearing in adolescence due to inflammation, with accumulation of secretions, involving the sebaceous glands.

Additives Elements added to natural foods not present originally.

Albumen or Albumin White of egg; proteins rich in sulphur and complex in structure.

Adrenal Of or from the adrenal glands; near or upon the kidneys.

Alkali Substance with properties of a base of hydroxide. Alkaline substances are soluble in water and can neutralize acid.

Allergy An abnormal or altered sensitivity to a specific substance (allergen).

177

Allopathy A system of treatment that seeks to cure a disease by producing a condition different from or incompatible with effects of the disease: opposed to homeopathy. —Allopathic.

Amino acids Any of a group of nitrogenous compounds that are structural units of protein and essential to the human metabolism.

Anemia A general or local deficiency in the amount of hemoglobin or number of red corpuscles in the blood, variously caused and characterized by pallor and loss of energy.

Antibodies Substances existing in the blood, either naturally or through deliberate immunization procedures, which counteract bacteria or bacterial poisons in the system.

Antidote Agent which counteracts or destroys the effects of poison or other medicine.

Aqueous chlorophyll Green pigment of plants deposited by water.

Arteriosclerosis The thickening and hardening of the inner walls of an artery, with impairment of blood circulation, as in old age.

Arthritis Inflammation of bone joints with resultant pain and disability.

Ascorbic acid Organic compound known as vitamin C, cevitamic acid and avitamic acid. Present in citrus fruits, tomatoes, strawberries and numerous other fruits.

Asthma Breathing difficulty due to an allergy to food or substances breathed into the system.

Atonic Without tone, loss or lack of tone.

Bacteria One-celled vegetable microorganisms containing no chlorophyll, which multiply by single division; concerned with fermentation and putrefaction.

Basal metabolism Minimal amount of energy or calories sufficient to support the basic metabolic processes of a person at rest, 12 hours after taking food.

Benign Not endangering health or life as opposed to malignant.

Betaine A crystalline alkaloid compound related to glycine found in the beet and various other plants.

Biochemistry Branch of chemistry relating to life processes, their modes of action and products.

Bioflavonoids Naturally occurring flavone or coumarin derivatives showing vitamin P activity, notably rutin and esculin.

Bile Bitter yellowish-brown or green fluid secreted by the liver serving to promote digestion. Aids in the emulsification of fats, increases peristalsis and retards putrefaction.

Bulk Vegetables such as carrots, cabbage, etc., containing "roughage" (cellulose) that increases the bulk of material in the intestine, thereby stimulating peristalsis.

Calcification Process in which tissue becomes hardened as a result of precipitates or larger deposits of insoluble salts of calcium.

Calcium Soft, silver-white metallic chemical element found in abundant quantities in the body: essential ingredient in bones and teeth. Found in milk products, beef, fish, vegetables, fresh fruits and nuts.

Calculus A stone-like mass, as in the bladder.—pl. calculi.

Calorie Amount of heat required to raise the temperature of one gram of water one degree centigrade. Used as a unit for measuring the energy produced by food when oxidized by the body.

Carbohydrates Certain organic compounds composed of carbon, hydrogen and oxygen; principal sources of food energy. Sugars, starches and cellulose are carbohydrates.

Carcinoma A malignant epithelial tumor that invades adjacent tissue and spreads by metastasis; cancer. Also carcinus.

Carminative Tending to, or used to, relieve flatulence. A remedy for flatulence.

Carotene A deep yellow or red crystalline hydrocarbon that acts as a plant pigment, especially in carrots, and occurs also in various animal tissues, when it is changed to vitamin A: also spelled carrotin, carotin.

Catalyst A small, often minute substance which accelerates or retards a chemical reaction but which does not in itself combine permanently with the resultant substances.

Cathartic Agent causing active movements of the bowels; laxative such as castor oil.

Cell A very small unit of protoplasm enclosed in a membrane and containing a nucleus: the living, active basis of all plant and animal life.

Cevitamic acid Ascorbic acid. (Synthetic).

Cholesterol Crystalline fatty alcohol found especially in animal fats, blood, nerve tissue and bile.

Cirrhosis Disease of the liver of unknown cause; interferes with liver function and circulation of blood and bile. Characterized by degeneration, fatty infiltration, atrophy and inflammation.

Climacteric An age or period of life characterized by marked physiological change, formerly believed to occur at ages that are multiples of seven and an odd number. —The menopause. —Any critical year or period.

Cobalamin Vitamin B-12.

Cobalt Hard, lustrous, steel-gray metallic element necessary for normal blood production.

Colitis Inflammation or spasm of large bowel often caused by emotional problems.

Collinsonia Herb also known as stone root.

Colon The portion of the large intestine between the cecum and the rectum.

Colonic Process of injecting a liquid into the colon to aid elimination.

Colloid Any glue-like or jelly-like substance as gelatin, starch, raw egg, etc. that diffuses not at all or very slowly through vegetables and animal membranes; distinguished from crystalloid.

Constipation Inability to perform normal bowel elimination function.

Contraindication Circumstances that indicate certain medical or surgical procedures should be avoided.

Corpuscle Any small mass or body; a blood cell.

Cortisone A powerful hormone extracted from the cortex of the adrenal gland and also made synthetically.

Crystalline Of, pertaining to, or like crystal or crystals— transparent; clear; pure. —Composed of crystal or crystals.

Deficiency disease A disease caused by the lack of essential constituents in the diet or by defective metabolism.

Dehydrate To remove moisture from foods; used to preserve foods.

Deleterious Causing moral or physical injury; hurtful.

Dentition The process or period of cutting teeth; teething.

Dermatitis Common name for skin irritation; inflammation of the dermis.

Dermis The corium or true skin, lying just below the epidermis or surface skin.

Detoxification The process of cleansing from toxins.

Digestion Process whereby ingested food is converted into material suitable for assimilation with the consequent buildup of tissues and liberation of energy in the body.

Digestive juices Secretions of the digestive system which act chemically to help convert food to forms the body can use.

Digitalis Basic drug for use in certain types of heart disease.

Diverticulitis Inflammation of the lower intestinal tract.

Dolomites A brittle calcium magnesium carbonate, occurring abundantly in white to pale pink rhombohedral crystals.

Ecology Scientific relationship between man and the other animals and plants and their environment.

Eczema Disease of the skin accompanied by inflammation, itching, water discharge and lesions.

Elimination Excretion of waste products from the body by the skin, kidneys and intestines.

Emollient Agent which softens or soothes skin or irritated internal surfaces.

Emphysema Respiratory system disease in which lung capacity is diminished and breathing efficiency impaired due to loss of elasticity in the muscles lining the bronchial system. Decreases the power of the lungs to expand. The use of tobacco, particularly cigarettes, and air pollution have contributed to the recent surge of emphysema conditions.

Empirical medicine Relying on practical experience without benefit of scientific knowledge or theory.

Endocrine The internal secretion of a gland—an endocrine gland.

Energy Vigor or intensity of action.

Enzymes Various proteins secreted by the body which act as catalysts in inducing chemical changes in other substances, particularly in digestion.

Ergosterol An inert sterol obtained from ergot, yeast, etc., and converted by irradiation of ultraviolet rays into calciferol.

Esophagus The tube in animals through which food passes from the mouth to the stomach; gullet; also spelled oesophagus.

Essential compounds Compounds synthesized by the body from the essential nutrients which are necessary for the maintenance of good health.

Essential fatty acids Fatty acids which must be furnished by the diet because the body cannot manufacture them.

Estrogen Any of various substances that influence estrus or produce changes in the sexual characteristics of female mammals, as estrone; also spelled oestrogen.

Excretions Wastes expelled from the body.

Fasting Abstaining from the intake of food.

Fat Oily or greasy soft-solid substances found in animal tissues and also occurring in certain plants and vegetables; an essential element in the diet to provide energy.

Fatigue Exhaustion; loss of energy; tiring as a result of physical or mental exertion.

Fat-soluble Class of substances in foods essential for growth and maintenance such as vitamins contained in butter and other animal fats which are capable of being dissolved in body fat.

Feces Animal excrement; ordure. —Any foul refuse matter or sediment.

Fermentation The gradual decomposition of organic compounds induced by the action of various ferments.

Flatulence An accumulation of gas in the intestinal tract.

Fluoridation Addition of fluorine salts to drinking water.

Fluorine Gaseous element not proven essential to life and subject to much controversy as to its importance in preventing cavities in the teeth.

Food values Relative nourishing power ascribed to foods.

Fortified Additions, e.g. vitamins, minerals, etc., made to a food product to give increased nutritional value.

Gamma globulin Protein substance found in blood serum; concerned with immunity against infections.

Gastrointestinal Of or pertaining to the stomach and intestines.

Geriatrics That branch of medicine which treats all problems peculiar to old age and the aging.

Germ Microscopic organism capable of causing disease.

Gland Any of various organs by means of which certain constituents are removed from the blood, either for use in the body or for elimination from it. Glands are of two types, those having ducts leading into another organ, as the pancreas, liver, etc., and those without ducts, as the adrenals, pituitary, etc., that pour their secretions directly into the bloodstream.

Globulin Any one of a group of simple plant and animal proteins, insoluble in water but soluble in dilute saline solutions.

Glucose A monosaccharide carbohydrate less sweet than cane sugar. It is widely distributed in the form of dextrose in plants and animals and is obtained by the hydrolysis of starch and other carbohydrates.

Gustatory Of or pertaining to the sense of taste or the act of tasting. Also gustative.

Health foods Foods eaten in their natural unprocessed state such as all whole-grained food, nuts, honey and unprocessed sugar.

Hemoglobin A protein; red coloring matter of the red blood corpuscles which carry oxygen from the lungs to the tissues and carbon dioxide from the tissues to the lungs.

Hesperidin A white, tasteless, odorless crystalline glycoside bioflavonoid obtained from citrus fruit.

Homeopathy A system of therapy using minute doses of medicines that produce the symptoms of the disease treated; opposed to allopathy. Also spelled homoeopathy.

Homogenize To make of uniform structure or composition throughout by breaking down and blending the different particles.

Homogeneous Having the same composition, structure or character throughout; uniform; a homogeneous mass.

Hormone Chemical substance formed in one organ or part of the body and carried to another organ or part which it stimulates to functional activity.

Hypertension High blood pressure.

Immunity Capacity of the body to resist infection.

Infection The invasion of the body tissues by disease-causing agents such as germs or fungi.

Infectious hepatitis Viral inflammation of the liver with evidence of jaundice.

Ingest To take into the body; to swallow.

Ingestion The act of taking food into the body for nourishment.

Inorganic Composed of inanimate matter.

Insoluble Incapable of being dissolved in a liquid.

Insulin A hormone in the pancreas which controls the level of blood sugar.

International Units (IU) Unit of measure applied to nutrients. Divide by 20 to convert units into milligrams.

Iodine Essential element for development of thyrosin which regulates the metabolism.

Ion An electrically charged atom, radical or molecule, produced by the dissolution of any electrolyte or by the actions of electric fields, high temperatures, various forms of radiation, etc., in adding or removing electrons.

Ionic Of or consisting of ions.

Iron Mineral vital to the functioning of the human body; aids in tissue respiration and in the formation of red corpuscles; helps carry oxygen to the blood.

Isometric exercise Physical exertion requiring the use of your full force against an immovable object.

Isotonics Exercises where muscle tension is combined with movement. The joints of the body move through a full range of motion against some form of resistance.

Jaundice A yellowish staining of the skin, deeper tissue and excretions with bile pigment; usually due to liver disturbance.

Kelp Any of various large coarse brown seaweed often used as a source of iodine in the diet.

Lactation The mammalian formation of secretion of milk. —The period during which milk is produced. —The act of suckling young.

Lactic acid Acid produced by the fermentation of milk sugar; accounts for the flavor of sour milk.

Lactose Milk sugar; white crystalline sugar found in milk.

Lanolin Hydrous wool fat used in ointments, cosmetics, soaps, etc. Purified wool fat used as emollient for the skin.

Laxative Preparation taken to produce evacuation of the bowels.

Lecithin Fatty substance found in blood, milk, egg yolk, nerve tissue and some vegetables and used as an emulsifier and aid to the assimilation of fat.

Leucine An essential amino acid.

Linolenic acid Unsaturated fatty acid essential in nutrition.

Lipolytic Pertaining to the decomposition of fats.

Lipotropic element Element in diet preventing abnormal or excessive accumulation of fat in the liver.

Live food Uncooked and unprocessed food.

Liver Largest and most important glandular organ. Vital to the digestive processes of both humans and animals, particularly in converting sugars for release into the bloodstream. As a food it is rich in vitamins A, B and C and iron.

Lymphatic Containing, conveying or pertaining to lymph. —Caused by or affecting the lymph nodes. —Sluggish, indifferent.

Lymphocytes A variety of nucleated, colorless leucocyte formed in the tissue of the lymph nodes and resembling white blood corpuscles.

Lysine An essential amino acid.

Magnesium oxide Fine white odorless powder insoluble in water; antacid and laxative.

Manganese A chemical element.

Manganese dioxide A compound formed from manganese.

Masticate To chew solid food in preparation for swallowing and digestion.

MDR—Minimum Daily Requirement Standard established as the lowest possible amount of a substance required by humans in order to avert a deficiency disease.

Metabolism The sum of the chemical changes whereby the function of nutrition is affected.

Methionine An essential amino acid.

Microorganism Minute living organism not perceptible to the naked eye.

Mineral Homogeneous inorganic material occurring naturally in the earth.

Mineral salts Inorganic salts including sodium, potassium, calcium, chloride, phosphate, sulfate, etc.

Mineral water Spring or well water containing carbon dioxide gas or salts or both; said to produce a tonic effect.

Molecule The smallest quantity into which a substance may be divided.

Multi-vitamin Having many vitamins.

Native Indigenous to a certain area (grown or produced naturally).

Natural vitamins Vitamins obtained from living, organic material as opposed to synthetic sources (formulated by mixing chemicals in a laboratory).

Naturopath A practitioner of healing who relies on natural methods to treat disease.

Nephritis Inflammation of the kidney.

Niacin Nicotinic acid; participates in a wide variety of metabolic processes; essential for functions of nervous system, soft tissue and liver.

Nitrite A salt of nitrous acid.

Nitrogen The chemical element in protein essential to human life; nitrogen is a gaseous element; odorless, colorless and tasteless.

Node A knot, knob, or swelling; protuberance.

Nourish To provide with food and sustenance.

Nutrient A substance that serves as nourishment.

Nutrition All foods; the physical processes by which food is converted into body tissue.

Nucleic acids Essential nutrients found within the nuclei of all living cells which constitute the very basis of life itself.

Obesity The condition of being fat.

Organic Coming from life; food grown without the use of chemical fertilizers or pesticides in soil made rich by composting and mulching; without the use of chemical sprays of any kind.

Organism Any living being.

Orthodox Adhering to traditional practice or belief; conventional; proper.

Orthophosphoric acid The common form of phosphoric acid, a colorless, syrupy liquid used in the manufacture of fertilizers.

Ovary The genital gland of female animals in which the essential reproductive elements or ova are produced.

Oxidation Process by which a substance is combined with oxygen.

Palliate To relieve the symptoms or effects of a disease, etc. without curing; alleviate; mitigate.

Pancreas A large gland situated behind the lower part of the stomach, secreting pancreatic juice into the duodenum.

Pancreatin A mixture of the enzymes contained in pancreatic juice; a preparation made from the fresh pancreas of hogs, cattle, etc. and used as a digestant.

Pasteurization The heating of milk for about 30 minutes at 60 degrees Centigrade, in order to destroy the living bacteria.

Pathologic Due to a disease.

Pectin Gelatinous substances present in fruits used in jellying fruit juices.

Pellagra Deficiency disease caused by improper diet and characterized by skin lesions, gastrointestinal disturbances and nervousness.

Pepsin An enzyme secreted by the gastric juices of the stomach that changes proteins into proteoses and peptones.

Peptic Pertaining to or aiding digestion.

Peristalsis Rhythmic contractions of the stomach.

pH Symbol used in expressing hydrogen ion concentration; the measure of alkalinity and acidity. pH 7 is the neutral point: above 7 alkalinity increases; below 7 acidity increases.

Phosphatase Group of enzymes that split the phosphate-carbohydrate compounds.

Phosphorus Mineral essential to the human body.

Pituitary Of or pertaining to the pituitary gland; produces internal secretions.

Placenta In higher mammals, the vascular, spongy organ of interlocking fetal and uterine membranes by which the fetus is nourished in the uterus. The part of the ovary that supports the ovules.

Potassium Element essential to human nutrition; important in maintaining the acid-base balance, the osmotic pressure and the health of nerves and muscles.

Potency The degree of power or strength, as of a drug.

ppm Parts per million.

Precursor One who or that which precedes, and suggests the course of future events; a substance from which another substance is formed.

Preservative Substance added to food products or organic solutions to preserve them from chemical change or bacterial action.

Preventive medicine Efforts to avoid the development of illness.

Protein One of a group of substances constituting the greater part of nitrogen-containing components of animal and vegetable tissues. An essential constituent of all living cells: for growth and development; for tissue maintenance and repair and healing; and recovery from disease.

Protein milk Acid milk with curd, richer in protein than ordinary milk and thought to be better tolerated in digestive disorders.

Proteolysis The change or splitting up of proteins into simpler products during digestion. Proteolytic.

Ptyalin An enzyme, contained in saliva, that converts starch into dextrin and maltose.

Ptyalism Abnormal flow of saliva; salivation.

Putrefaction The progressive chemical decomposition of organic matter, with the production of foul-smelling compounds. The state of being putrefied.

Pyridoxine Vitamin B-6, a water-soluble compound occurring in cereal grains, vegetable oils, legumes, yeast, meats and fish; also made synthetically.

Rancid Spoiled; having an unpleasant taste, especially as applied to butter and oils.

Raw milk Not pasteurized; in its natural state; not changed or prepared by heating.

Raw sugar Brown unrefined sugar 96 to 98 percent pure.

Regeneration Repair, regrowth or restoration of a part.

Regimen A program, as of healthful living.

Respiration The total process by which oxygen is absorbed into the system and the oxidation products such as carbon dioxide and water are given off.

Riboflavin A member of the vitamin B complex (B-2); an orange-yellow, crystalline compound found in milk, leafy vegetables, egg yolk and meats; also made synthetically.

Rutin Bioflavonoid obtained from buckwheat and having an action similar to that of vitamin P; causes increased capillary resistance.

Saliva The slightly alkaline fluid containing ptyalin and secreted by the glands of the mouth, considered as promoter of digestion. Salivary.

Salt Sodium chloride; ordinary table salt obtained from salt deposits, sea water, etc. Also refers to a compound formed by the interaction of an acid and a base.

Salt-free diets Those diets in which no salt has been added to foods. Required in cases of hypertension and cardiac insufficiency accompanied by edema, nephritis and nephrosis to reduce the fluid in the body.

Saline Salty; containing salt.

Secretion The process, generally a glandular function by which materials are separated from the blood and elaborated into new substances, as bile, saliva, milk, etc. A product of the process.

Slant board Board large enough to hold an adult, constructed in such a way that the head is almost to the ground and the feet are elevated; used to aid in normalizing circulation and in exercise.

Sodium An element essential in the human body.

Sodium chloride Ordinary table salt; a dietary essential usually satisfied by the normal nutritious diet.

Soluble Capable of being dissolved; water soluble, in water; fat soluble, in fats or oils.

Spleen A gland-like organ found near the stomach of every animal.

Starch Tasteless white substance found in various foods, such as potatoes, beans, corn, etc., source of fuel for the body.

Supplement A nutrient which is added to supply that which is lacking or to reinforce a product.

Synergistic Acting together; cooperative. Also synergistical.

Synthesized The process of building a product within the body from separate elements.

Therapeutic In this book, that branch of nutrition concerned with the treatment of disease.

Thiamine A white crystalline compound vitamin B-1, found in various natural sources; also made synthetically. Important for the health of the nervous system.

Thymus A glandular organ of man and some other vertebrates, found behind the top of the sternum, most prominent in youth and believed to influence immunity.

Tissue A collection of similar cells and the intercellular substances surrounding them.

Tocopherol Any of a group of alcohols having the properties of vitamin E; main source is wheat germ oil. There are four tocopherols and all possess vitamin E activity: alpha, beta, gamma and delta.

Toxemia Distribution through the body of poisonous products of bacteria which grow in a focal site.

Toxins Poisons.

Trichina A small nematode worm, parasitic in the intestines and muscles of man, swine and other mammals. pl. trichinae.

Varicose A dilated portion of a vein.

Villus One of the short, hairlike processes found on certain membranes, as of the small intestine, where they aid in the digestive process. One of the long, close, rather soft hairs on the surface of certain plants Pl. villi.

Viosterol Irradiated ergosterol, a vitamin D preparation variously used in tablets etc.

Vitamins Two general classes: the fat-soluble (vitamins A, D, E and K) and the water-soluble B-complex and C varieties. Many vitamins are depleted or destroyed by exposure to light, air, heat or alkaline conditions. They are therefore often lost from food through improper storage or cooking.

Vitamin B complex Consists of at least eight separate essential vitamins; originally thought to be only one. Although they perform different functions, they seem to act somewhat synergistically. They occur in many of the same foods; the richest sources are liver, whole grains, yeast and unpolished rice. The vitamins are necessary for efficient metabolism. Deficiencies often occur that involve several of these vitamins simultaneously.

The Best in Health Books by
LINDA CLARK,
BEATRICE TRUM HUNTER
and CARLSON WADE

By Linda Clark

☐ **Know Your Nutrition**
☐ **Cloth $5.95** ☐ **Paperback $3.50**
☐ **Face Improvement Through Exercise and**
   Nutrition   **$1.75**
☐ **Be Slim and Healthy**   **$1.50**
☐ **Go-Caution-Stop Carbohydrate Computer**   **95ᶜ**
☐ **Light on Your Health Problems**   **$1.25**
☐ **The Best of Linda Clark**   **$3.50**

By Beatrice Trum Hunter

☐ **Whole Grain Baking Sampler**
☐ **Cloth $6.95** ☐ **Paperback $2.25**
☐ **Food Additives and Your Health**   **$1.25**
☐ **Fermented Foods and Beverages**   **$1.25**
☐ **Golden Harvest Prize Winning Recipes**
   (ed. by BTH)   **$1.25**
☐ **Food and Your Health** (Anthology ed. by BTH) **$1.25**

By Carlson Wade

☐ **Fats, Oils and Cholesterol**   **$1.50**
☐ **Vitamins and Other Supplements**   **$1.25**
☐ **Hypertension (High Blood Pressure)**
   and Your Diet   **$1.50**
Buy them at your local health or book store or use this coupon.

Keats Publishing, Inc. (P.O. Box 876), New Canaan, Conn. 06840   75-A
Please send me the books I have checked above. I am enclosing
$_____ (add 35ᶜ to cover postage and handling). Send check or
money order—no cash or C.O.D.'s please.
Mr/Mrs/Miss_____

Address _____

City _____ State _____ Zip_____
          (Allow three weeks for delivery)

COOKBOOKS ON NATURAL HEALTH
. . . To Help You Eat Better for Less!

☐ **ADD A FEW SPROUTS** (Martha H. Oliver) **$1.50**

☐ **WHOLE GRAIN BAKING SAMPLER**
  (Beatrice Trum Hunter) **$2.25**

☐ **MRS. APPLEYARD'S KITCHEN** (L.A. Kent) **$3.50**

☐ **MRS. APPLEYARD'S SUMMER KITCHEN**
  (L.A. Kent & E.K. Gay) **$3.50**

☐ **MRS. APPLEYARD'S WINTER KITCHEN**
  (L.A. Kent & E.K. Gay) **$3.50**

☐ **BETTER FOODS FOR BETTER BABIES** (Gena Larson) **$1.25**

☐ **GOOD FOODS THAT GO TOGETHER** (Elinor L. Smith) **$2.95**

☐ **MEALS AND MENUS FOR ALL SEASONS** (Agnes Toms) **$1.25**

☐ **NATURAL FOODS BLENDER COOKBOOK**
  (Frieda Nusz) **$1.50**

☐ **GOLDEN HARVEST PRIZE WINNING RECIPES**
  (ed. by B.T. Hunter) **$1.25**

☐ **SOYBEANS FOR HEALTH** (Philip Chen) **$1.50**

☐ **FOOD AND FELLOWSHIP** (Elizabeth S. Pistole) **95ᶜ**

☐ **MENNONITE COMMUNITY COOKBOOK**
  (Mary Emma Showalter) **$1.25**

☐ **EAT THE WEEDS** (Ben Charles Harris) **$1.50**

Buy them at your local health or book store or use this coupon.

Keats Publishing, Inc. (P.O. Box 876), New Canaan, Conn. 06840 75-G
Please send me the books I have checked above. I am enclosing
$____ (add 35ᶜ to cover postage and handling). Send check or
money order—no cash or C.O.D.'s please.

Mr/Mrs/Miss_____

Address _____

City _____State _____Zip_____
(Allow three weeks for delivery)